'Help! I've got a voice problem'
by Lydia Hart and Stephen R King

art and design by Stewart Harris

'This wonderfully accessible book emphasises the many and various ways in which voices can go wrong. In discussing biological, psychological and sociological factors, it helps readers to understand that there is rarely just one factor causing vocal dysfunction. A fabulous introduction to voice disorders.'

— Declan Costello, Consultant ENT Surgeon specialising in voice disorders

Lydia is a Speech and Language Therapist who specialises in integrated therapy for voice, mind and body.

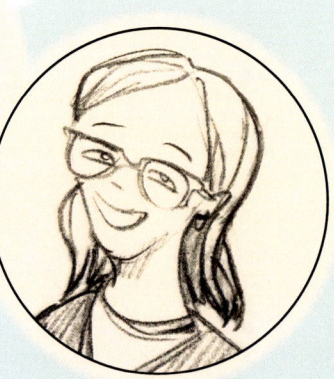

Stephen is a thought leader, educator and interdisciplinary therapist working in the field of voice health.

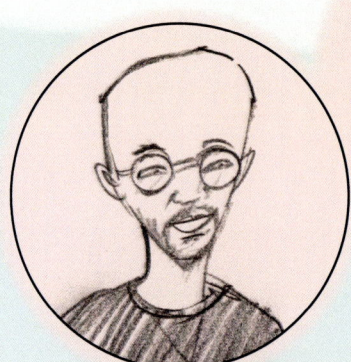

Stewart is an illustrator and graphic designer who is passionate about tea and biscuits.

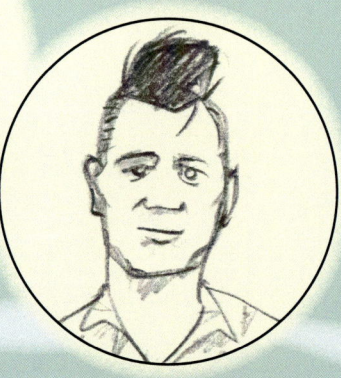

This book is dedicated to everyone without a voice

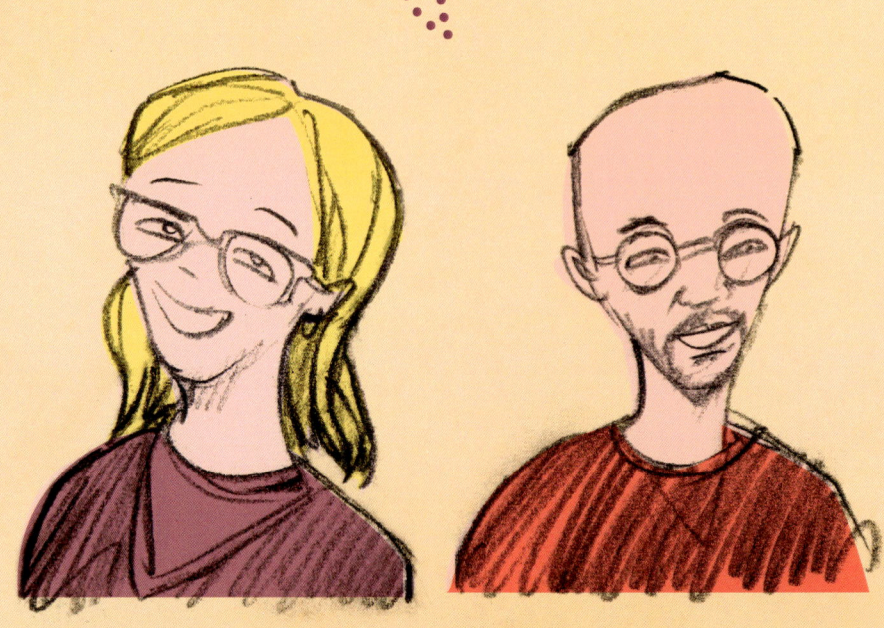

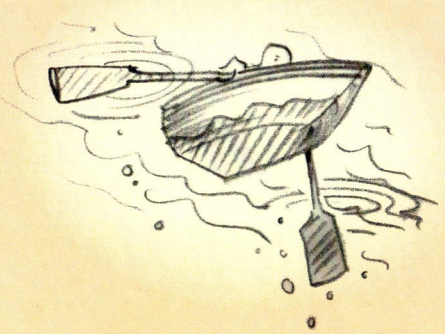

'Something's not right with my voice'

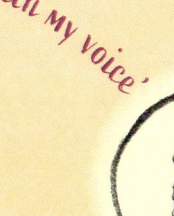

Page 6

OK, so I think there's something wrong, but what do I do?

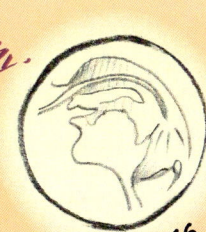

Page 12

'At this point, it is useful to remind ourselves of anatomy'

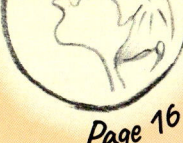

Page 16

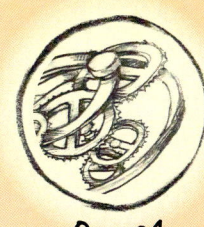

Page 21

'Our voice is part of a system'

'Let's return to our pathway to recovery'

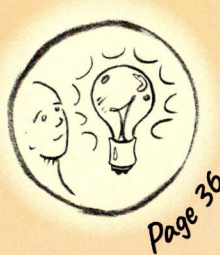

Page 29

'So what can I do to help myself?'

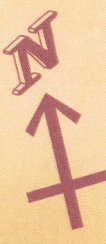

Page 36

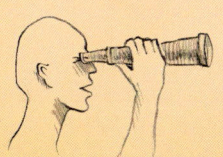

References
Page 44

"Something's not right with my voice..."

First of all, *it's not your fault*. There are lots of factors that make up any dysfunction* in the body, especially when it comes to the voice.

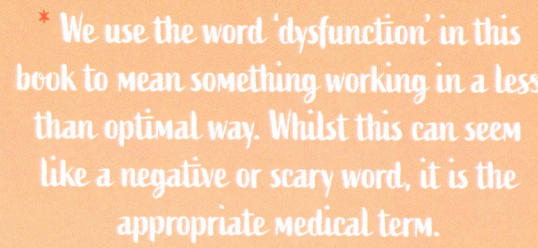

Like with any complex system, sometimes things can go wrong. Some people will recover quickly whereas for others it can be a longer road.

* We use the word 'dysfunction' in this book to mean something working in a less than optimal way. Whilst this can seem like a negative or scary word, it is the appropriate medical term.

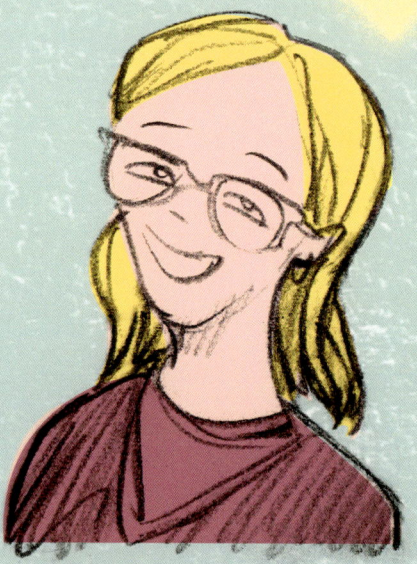
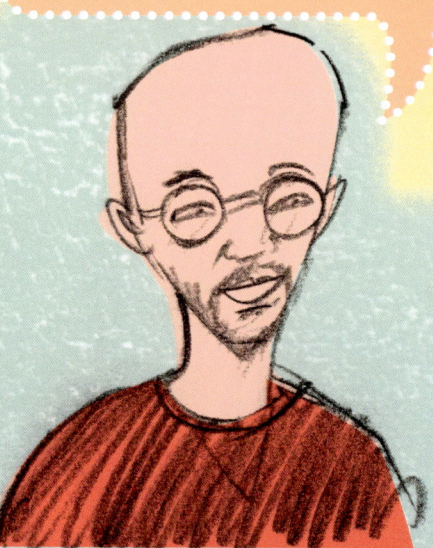

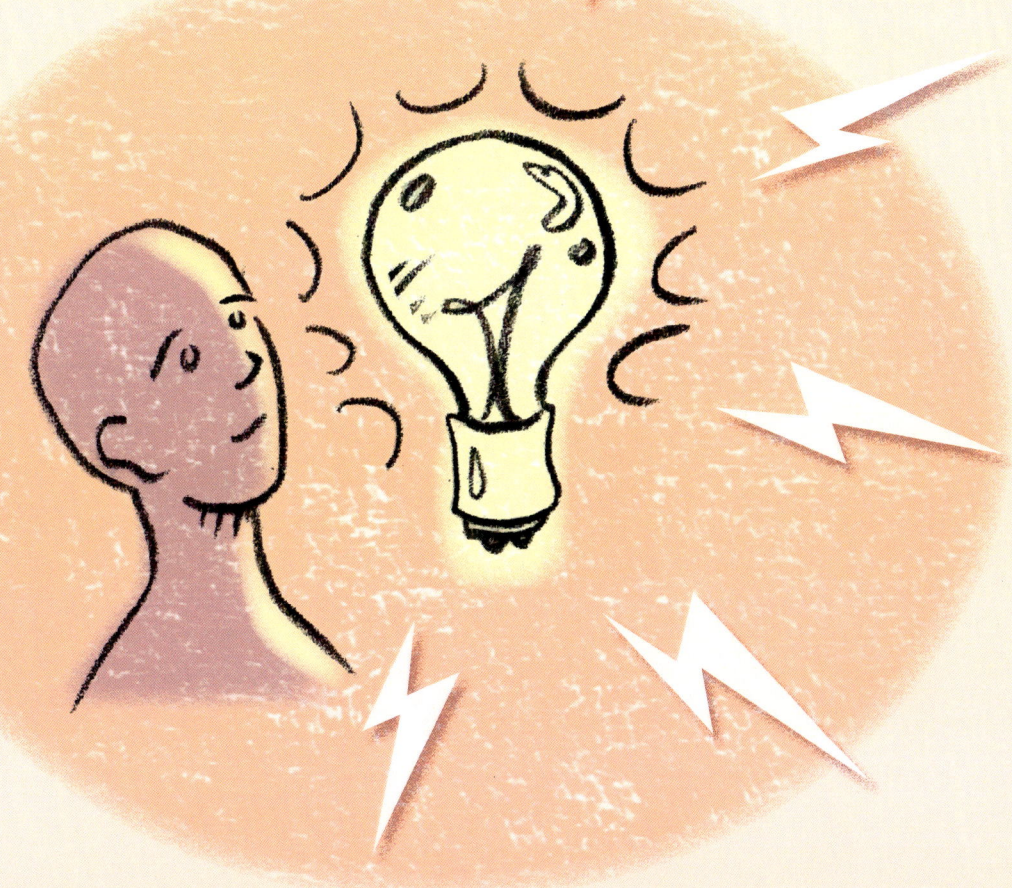

This book will help you to understand why you may have a voice problem, and what recovery could look like.

Your voice, and its home in your throat, is amazing. This home, which is called your *larynx*, is made of many muscles, membranes and cartilages, which are connected to your *brain* by *nerves*.

This allows you to...

Breathe
Cough
Swallow
Speak
Sing!

This wonderful, complex mechanism allows you to communicate with the world, but actually, *the main purpose of this mechanism is to keep you alive!*

In order to function optimally, all those muscles and nerves have to be working in balance, with your brain as the command centre.

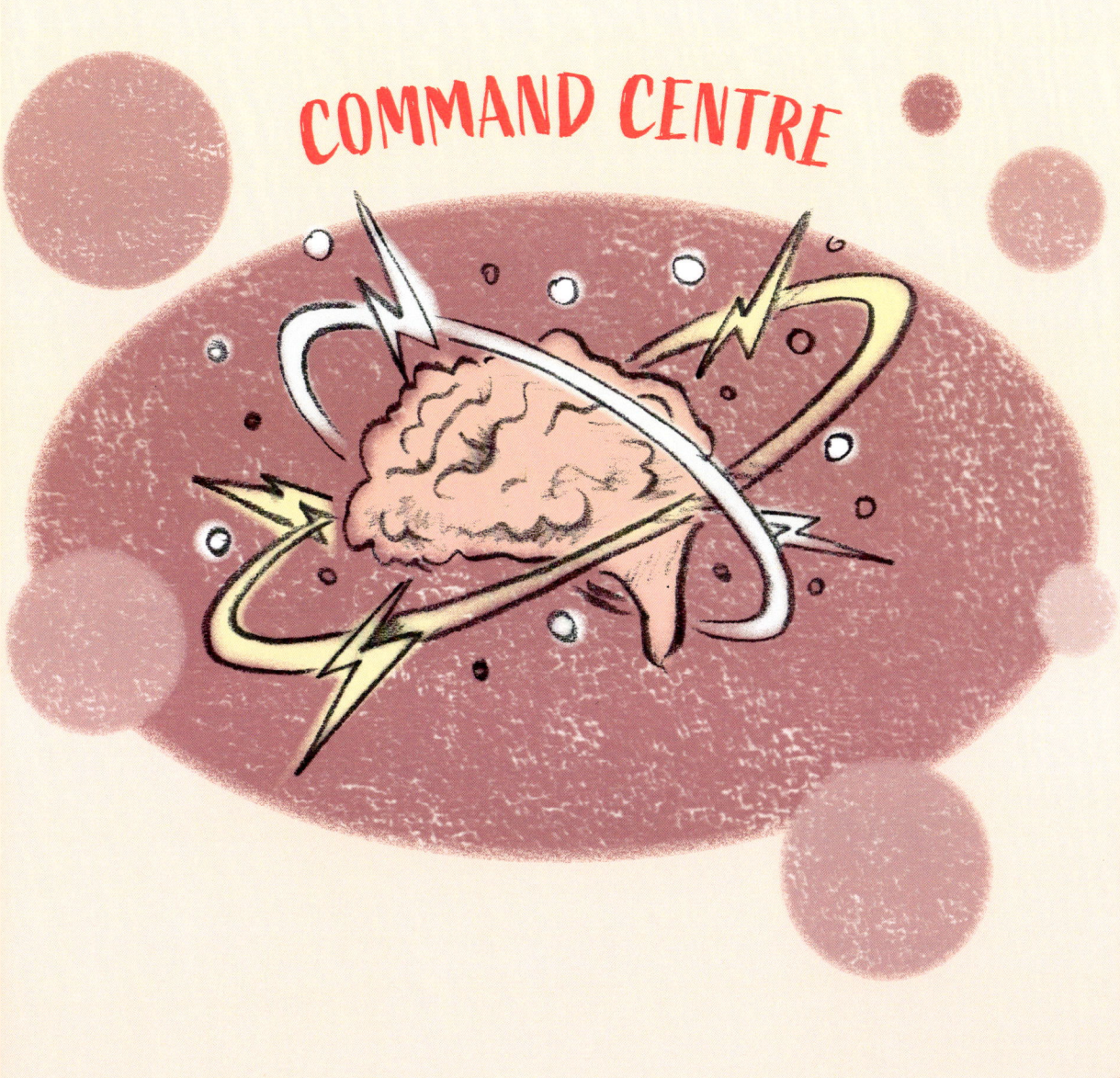

COMMAND CENTRE

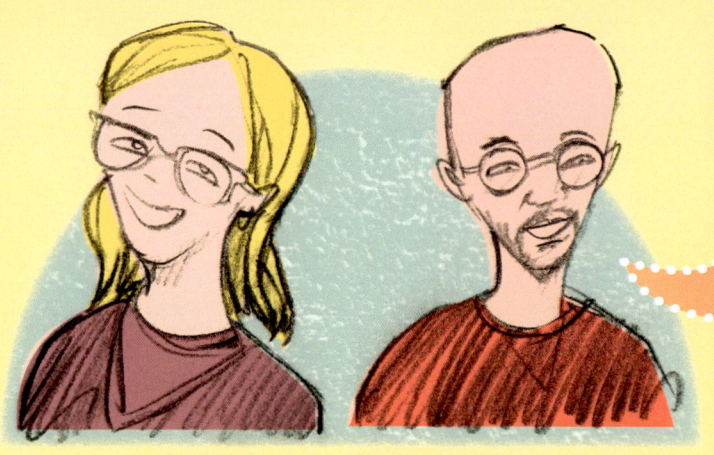

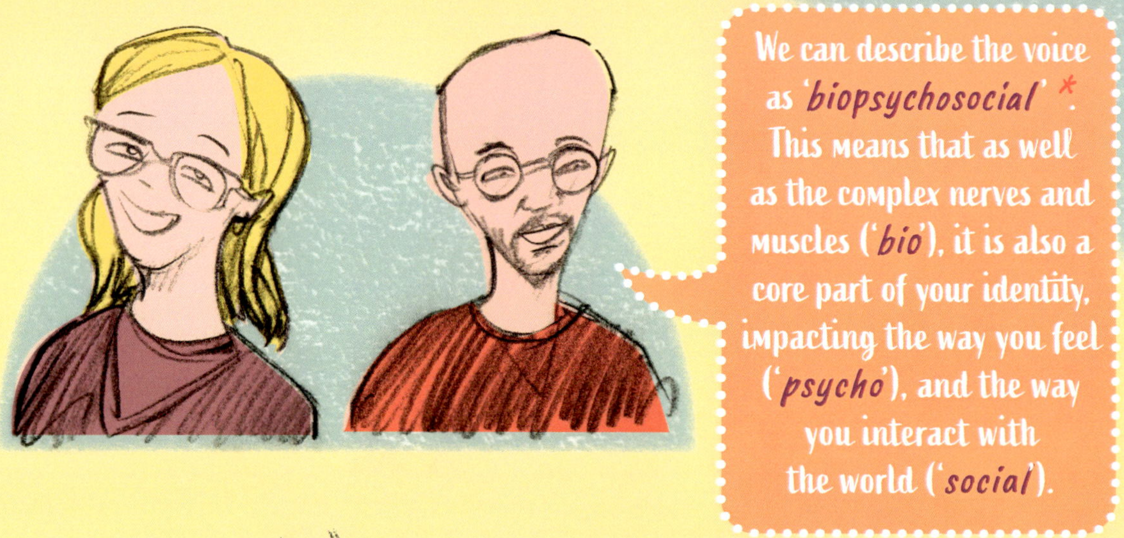

We can describe the voice as *'biopsychosocial'* *. This means that as well as the complex nerves and muscles (*'bio'*), it is also a core part of your identity, impacting the way you feel (*'psycho'*), and the way you interact with the world (*'social'*).

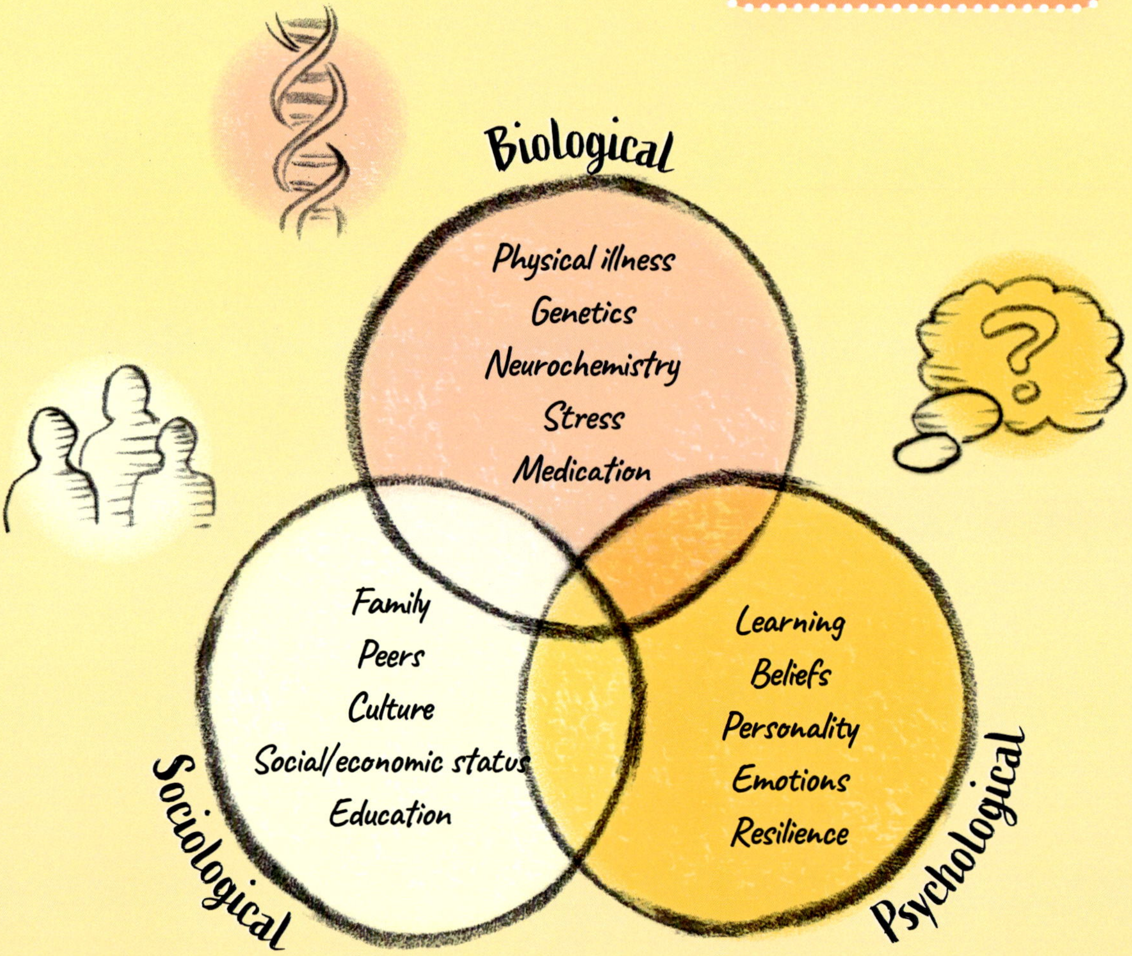

Biological
- Physical illness
- Genetics
- Neurochemistry
- Stress
- Medication

Sociological
- Family
- Peers
- Culture
- Social/economic status
- Education

Psychological
- Learning
- Beliefs
- Personality
- Emotions
- Resilience

*There are lots of different philosophies of medicine and approaches to understanding dysfunction and healing. The *Biopsychosocial Model*, and the *Evidence Based Model* are the two leaders in the field.

Because your voice is biopsychosocial, this can affect your work life, relationships and social activities, your mental health and even how you believe people perceive you.

It's how these three biopsychosocial parts *interact* which gives us a journey to recovery.

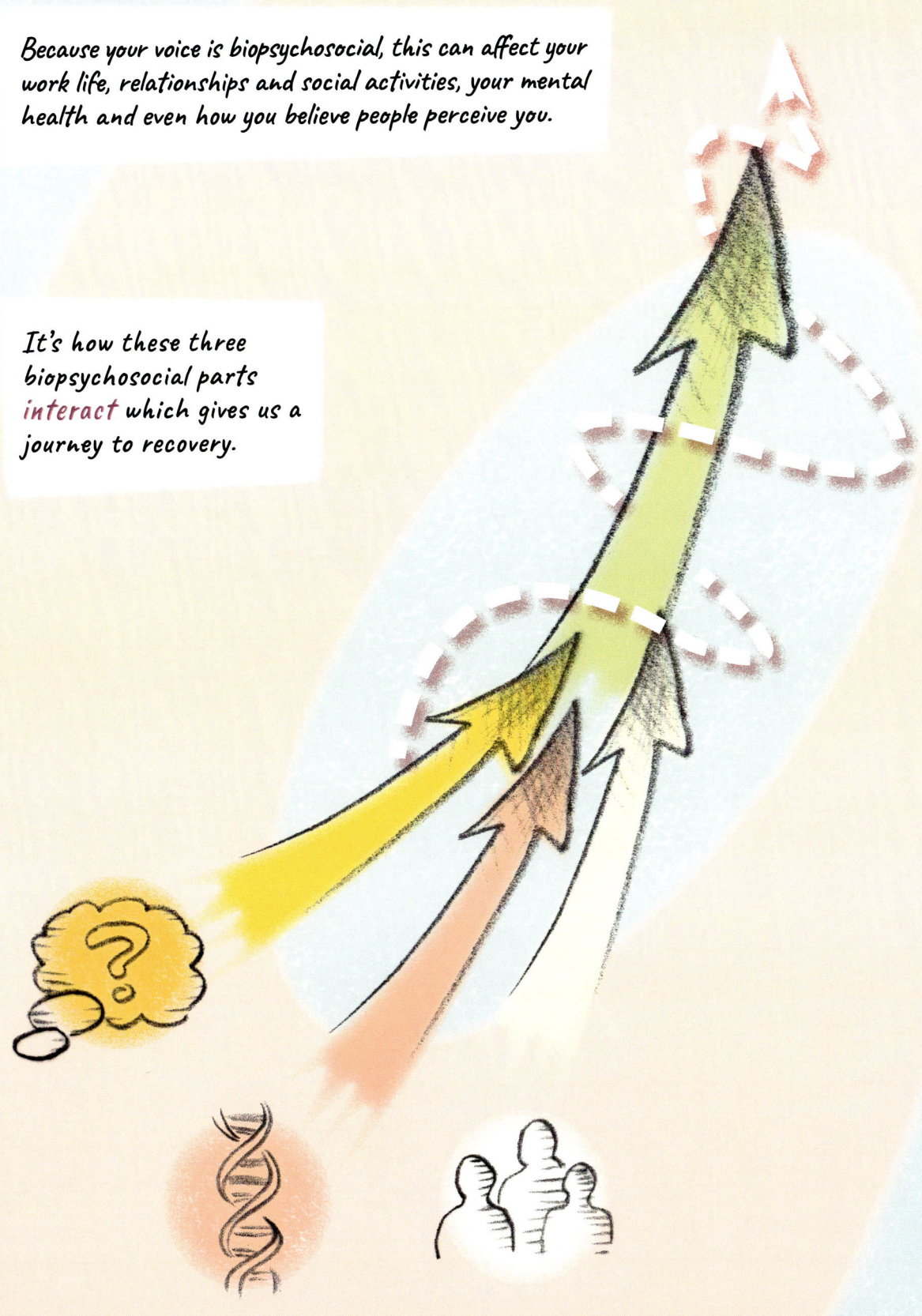

"OK, so I think there's something wrong, but what do I do?"

Throat problems are relatively common. 'Globus', which is the feeling of a lump in your throat, is experienced by around **40%** of people at some point in their lives.

If you are experiencing throat symptoms (such as hoarseness, pain, or globus) for more than three weeks, then it is a good idea to see a doctor because there may be a medical component that needs investigation and treatment.

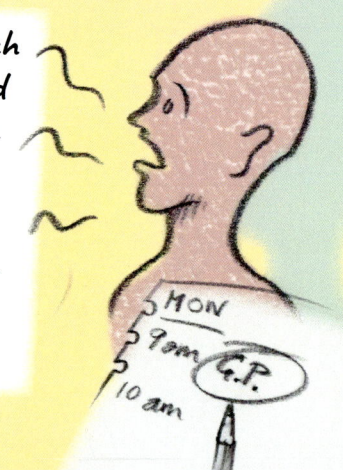

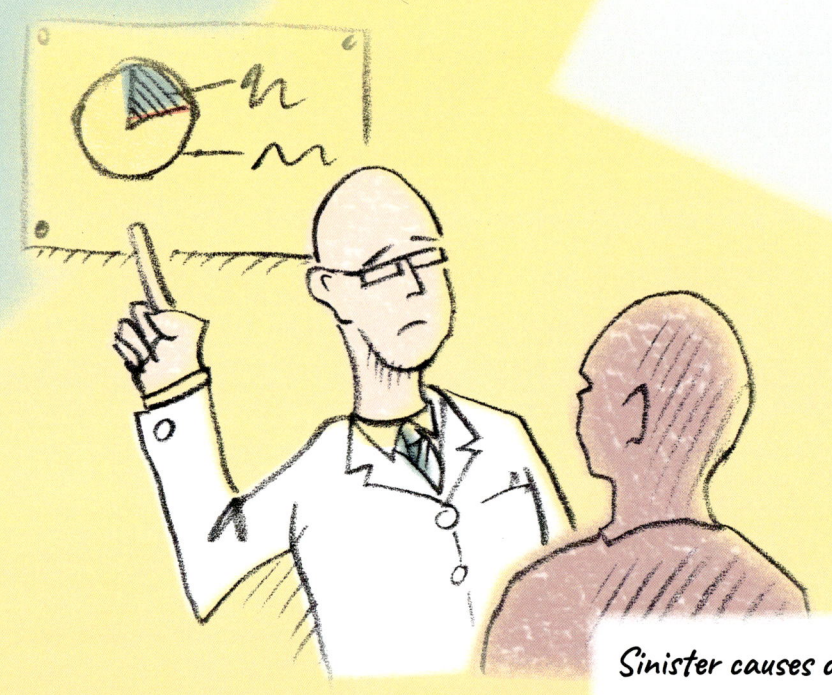

Sinister causes of throat symptoms are rare – only around **3%** of cases are caused by cancer*.

*Yikes! The c-word. But it is worth mentioning here, because it's one of the first things Doctors want to rule out when treating voice problems.

There can be lots of reasons why we might see a doctor, and sometimes – due to the complex overlapping of symptoms – there isn't a diagnosis that can be given straight away.

20% Medically unexplained symptoms (MUS)

3% Cancer

Other confirmed diagnosis

In the UK for example, **20%** of all General Practitioner (GP) appointments are people with Medically Unexplained Symptoms (MUS)*.

It's OK for the GP not to know what your symptoms mean, as they work with many different aspects of health and illness. This is why a referral to a specialist is needed.

*By the way: MUS is now a financial epidemic with an estimated cost to the UK's NHS of £3.1billion per year (of a total £18billion spent). In Germany (2013), the MUS figure in primary care was thought to be a massive 66%. So there is a likelihood your GP may not know what your symptoms mean.

Whilst it is important to see your doctor, it is likely that you may not get the answers you need straight away. This is because:

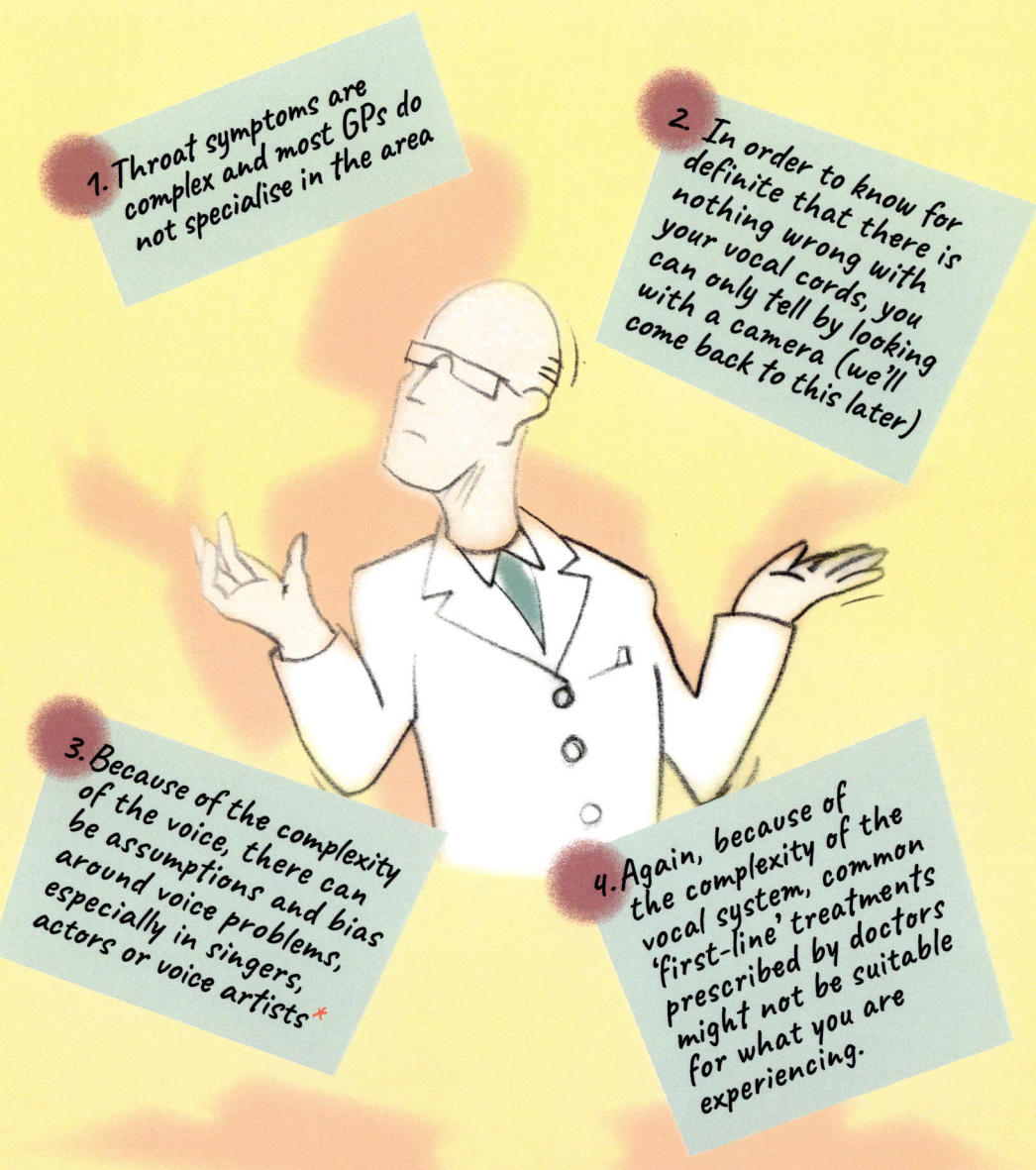

1. Throat symptoms are complex and most GPs do not specialise in the area

2. In order to know for definite that there is nothing wrong with your vocal cords, you can only tell by looking with a camera (we'll come back to this later)

3. Because of the complexity of the voice, there can be assumptions and bias around voice problems, especially in singers, actors or voice artists*

4. Again, because of the complexity of the vocal system, common 'first-line' treatments prescribed by doctors might not be suitable for what you are experiencing.

*People who work in the performing arts use their voices in highly skilled and specialist ways, and therefore experience vocal dysfunction differently than the rest of the population. It can be difficult for frontline medical practitioners to understand the impact this has, or know how to help, and this means performers can feel that they have been dismissed, or not listened to.

When you see a doctor, these are some things they may say is the cause of your voice problems:
- Reflux
- Laryngitis
- An infection
- Vocal abuse
- Nasal problems

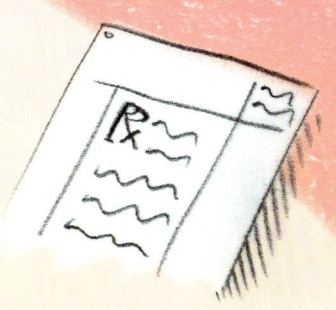

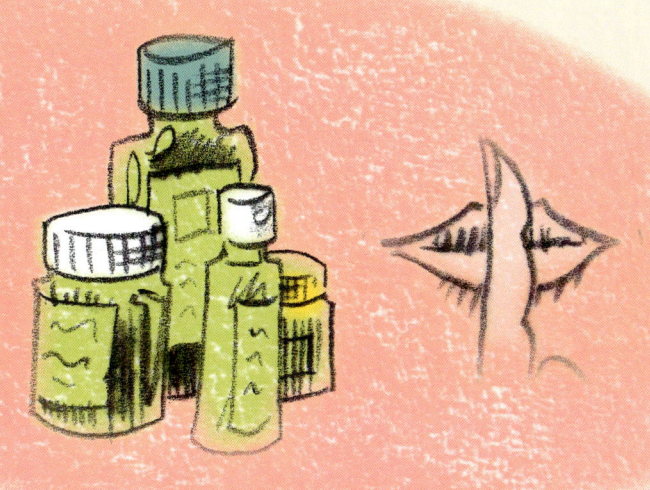

They may put you on the following treatments:
- Reflux tablets
- Antibiotics
- Voice rest
- Nasal sprays

If any of these treatments or prescriptions work, fantastic!

However if these don't work, you may be left feeling confused, frustrated or let down. These feelings, and the mindset they can cause, can make your symptoms worse.

Understanding the impact our emotions have on the voice is something we will come back to later.

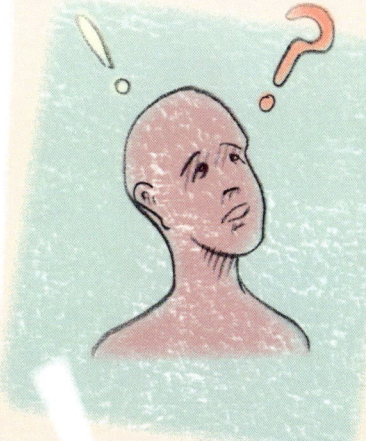

"At this point, it is useful to remind ourselves of anatomy..."

Let's have a brief look at the anatomy involved in our voice and breathing.

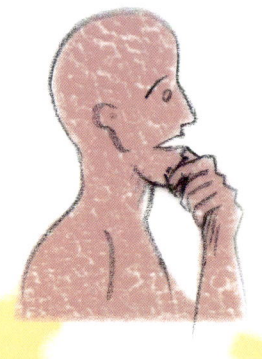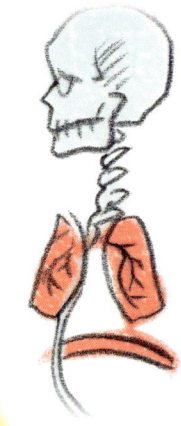

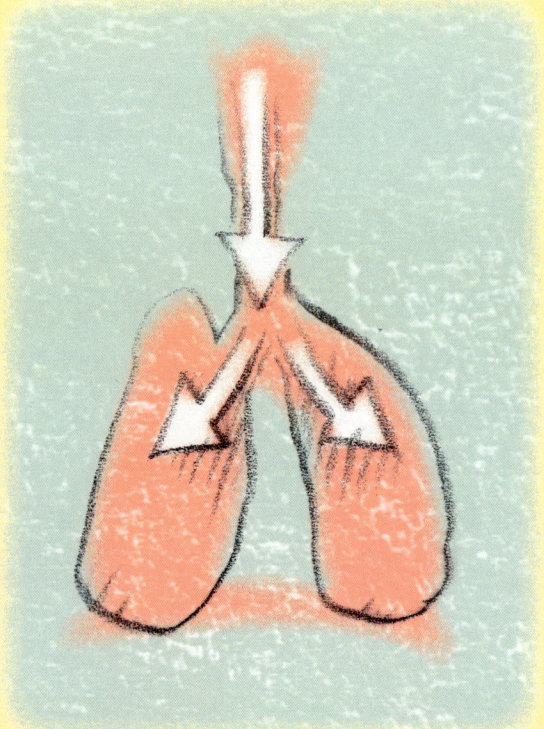

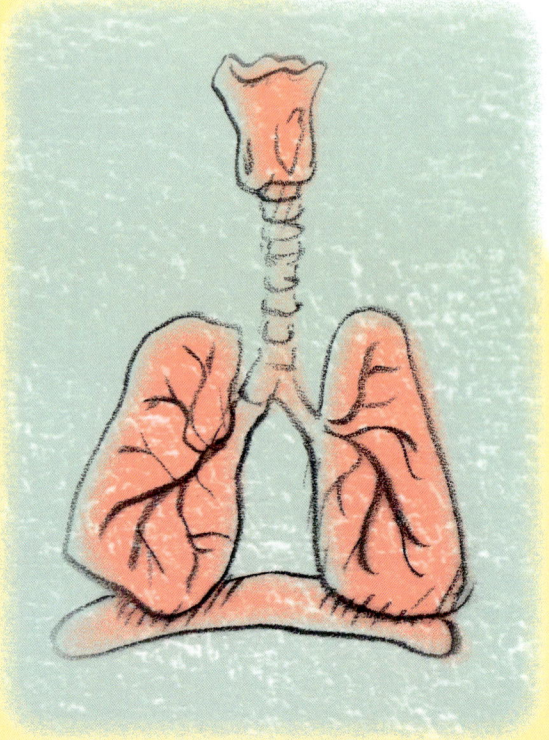

To breathe in, air is pulled into the lungs by the diaphragm (as well as the muscles between the ribs).

The diaphragm is a thin, dome shaped muscle that sits underneath the lungs. When the diaphragm activates, it pulls down into the abdominal cavity.

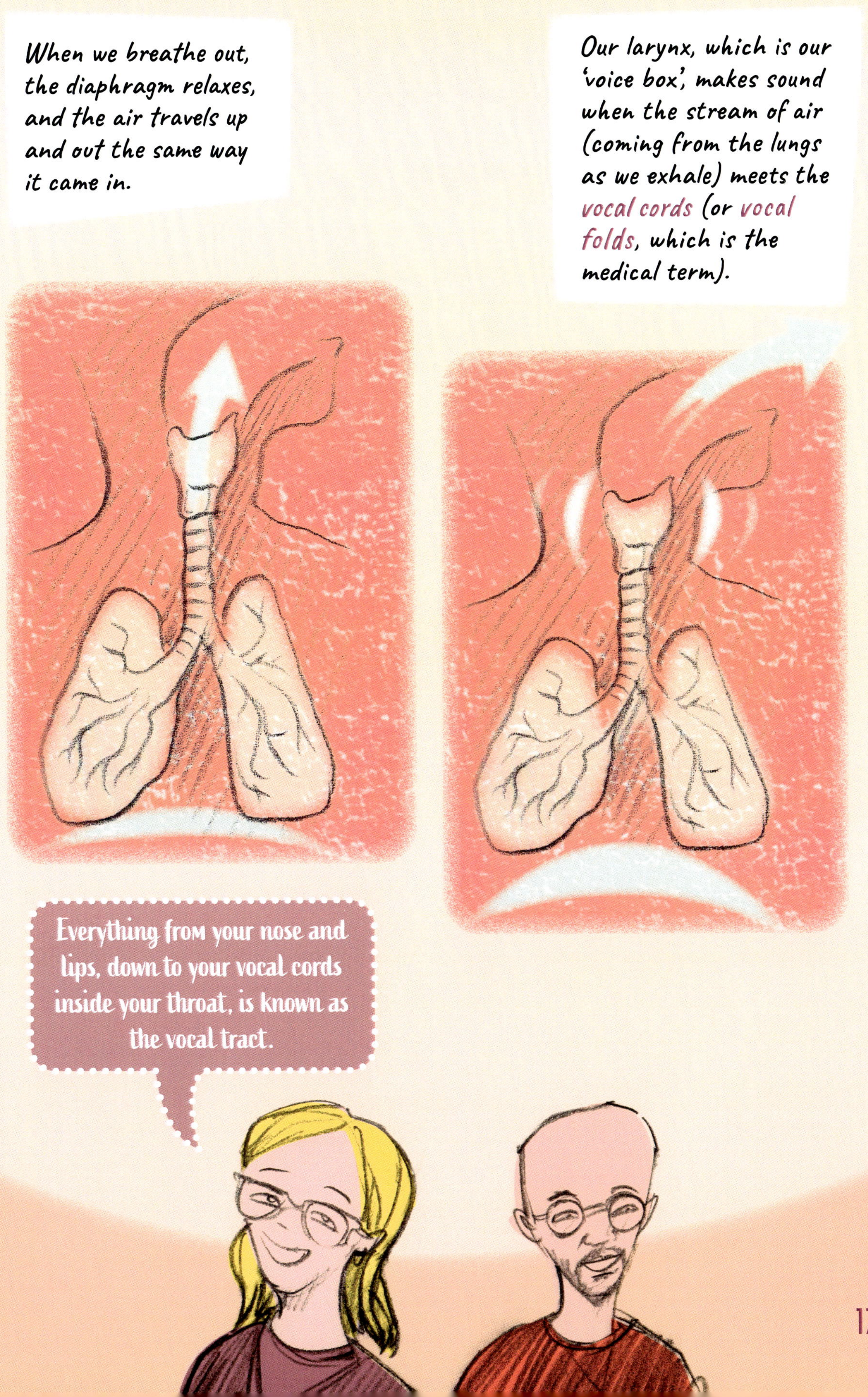

When we breathe out, the diaphragm relaxes, and the air travels up and out the same way it came in.

Our larynx, which is our 'voice box', makes sound when the stream of air (coming from the lungs as we exhale) meets the *vocal cords* (or *vocal folds*, which is the medical term).

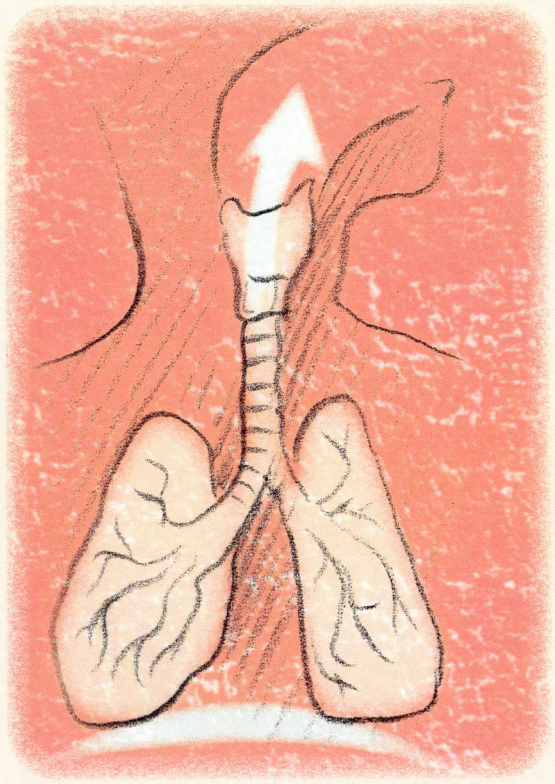

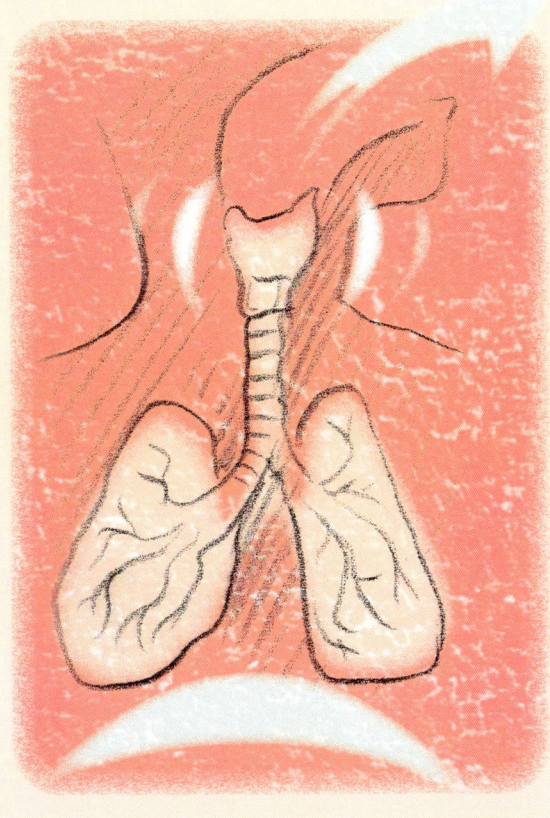

Everything from your nose and lips, down to your vocal cords inside your throat, is known as the vocal tract.

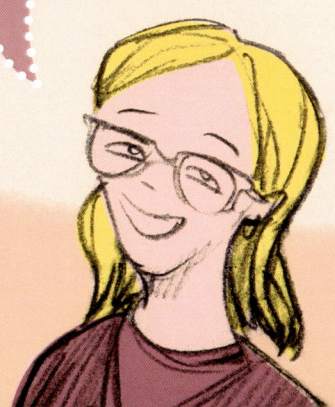

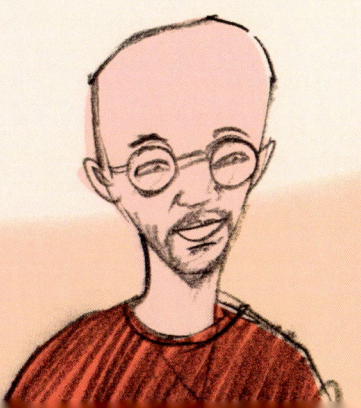

When we are breathing normally, our vocal cords sit apart in a 'V' shape, and the air passes through.

When we speak or sing (as well as when we swallow, cough, sneeze, or hold our breath!) the vocal cords close together.

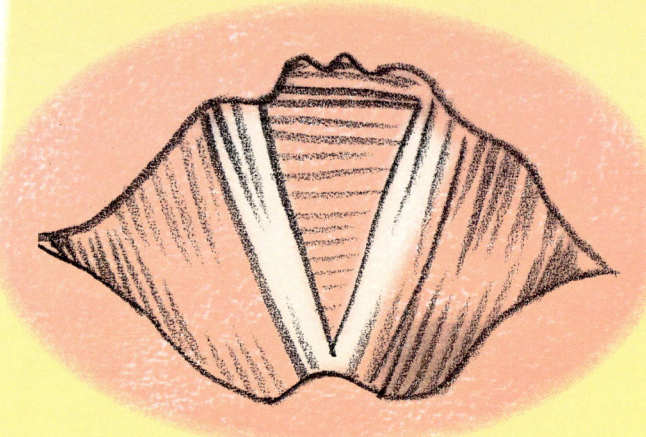

You can test this out right now - breathe in, hold your breath, then release your breath in a 'pop'. That's your vocal cords closing and opening!

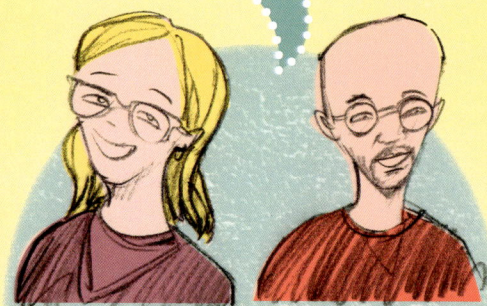

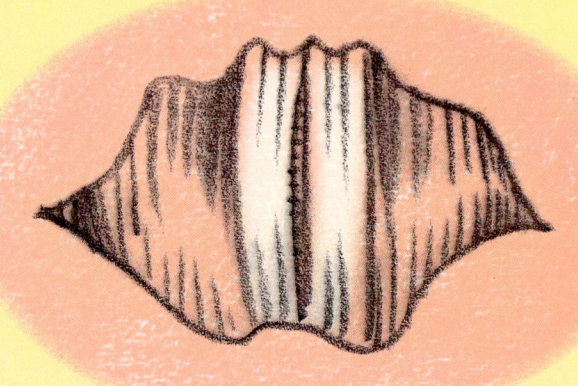

When the air meets the closed vocal cords, they vibrate. More specifically, they are sucked together and blown apart in an 'oscillatory' pattern. Sometimes (depending on the frequency*) this cycle of vibration can be over a thousand times per second!

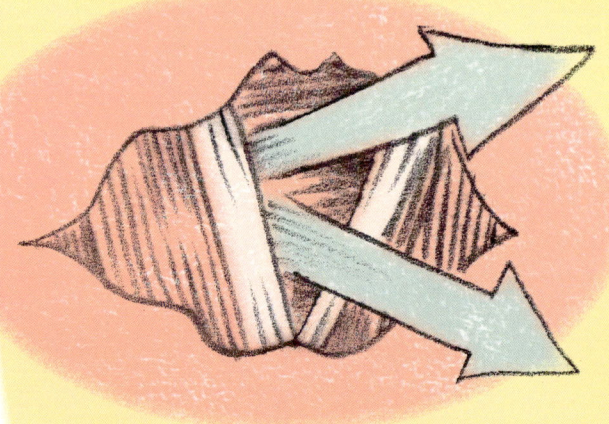

*The frequency is essentially the speed at which your vocal cords are vibrating (measured by the number of collisions of the cords per second), which determines the pitch of the sound.

Let's take a look at the vocal tract in a bit more detail...

Your *larynx* is a group of cartilages (and one bone) that are connected by muscles and membranes. The vocal cords sit in the middle of the biggest cartilage, the *thyroid* cartilage, and are moved by some of the smaller muscles.

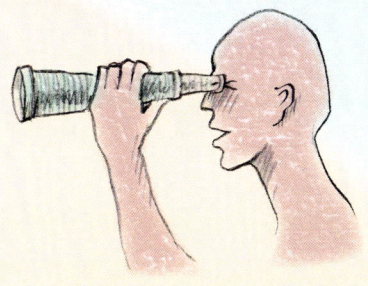

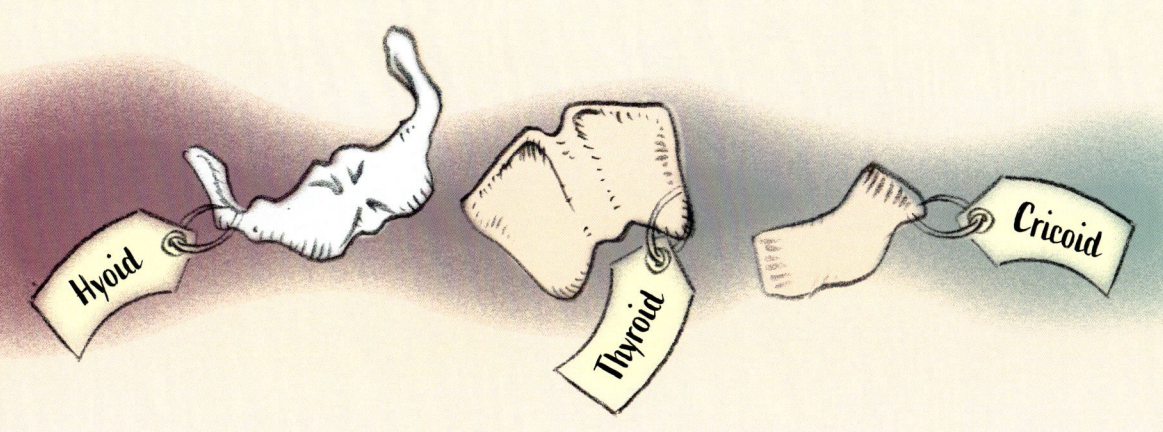

There are also long thin muscles, called *strap muscles*, which hold the larynx in place in your neck by connecting it to other structures.

Above the vocal cords is the rest of the vocal tract, which includes structures such as your *tongue*, *soft palate* and *lips*. These bits of our anatomy 'filter' and shape the sounds we make, by changing position as we speak and sing.

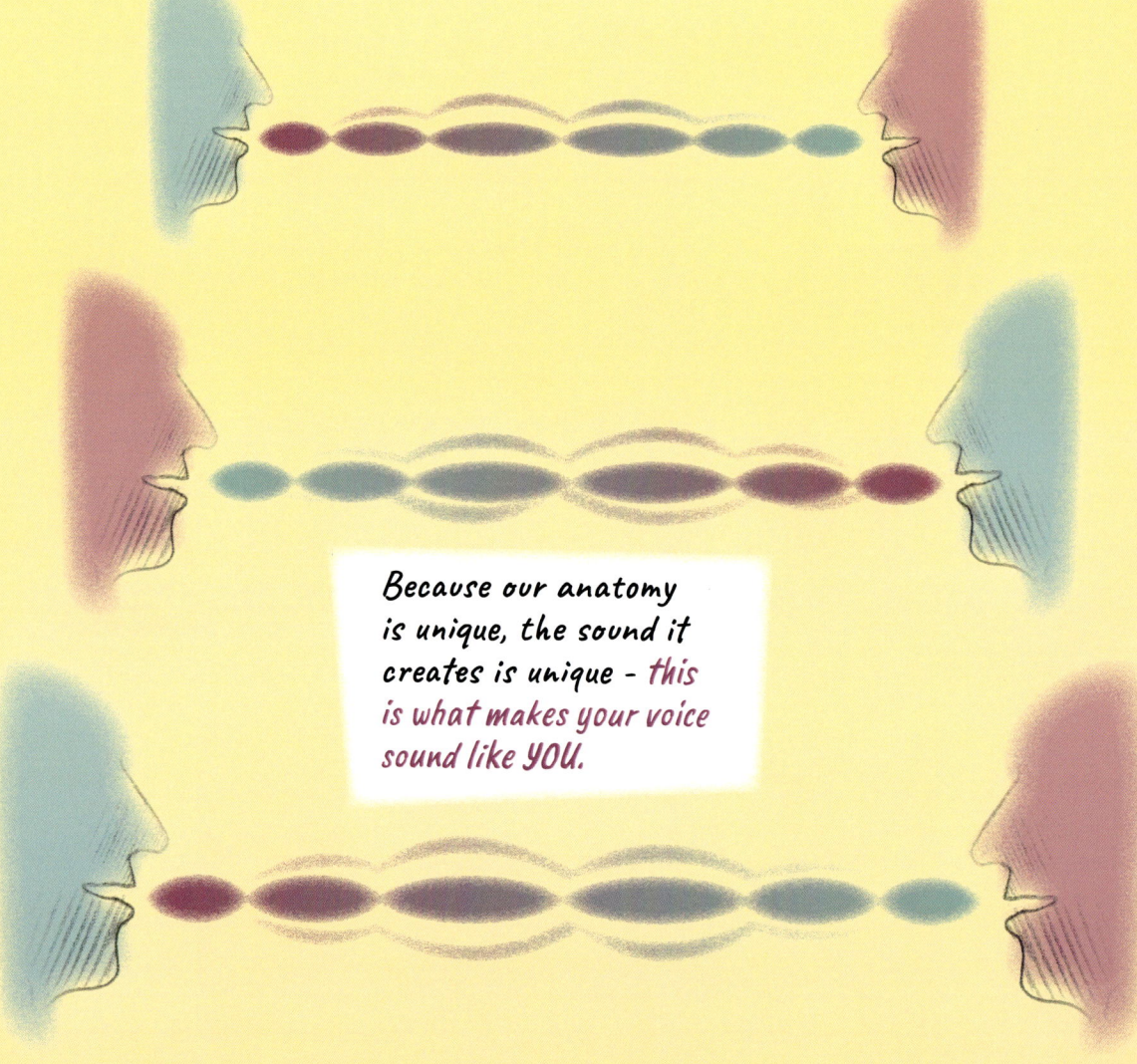

Because our anatomy is unique, the sound it creates is unique - *this is what makes your voice sound like YOU.*

"Our voice is part of a system"

The larynx is very sensitive to our emotions. If you were on the phone to a friend who was upset, (or angry, excited or afraid), you would be able to tell how they are feeling from the sound of their voice.

Isn't that amazing?

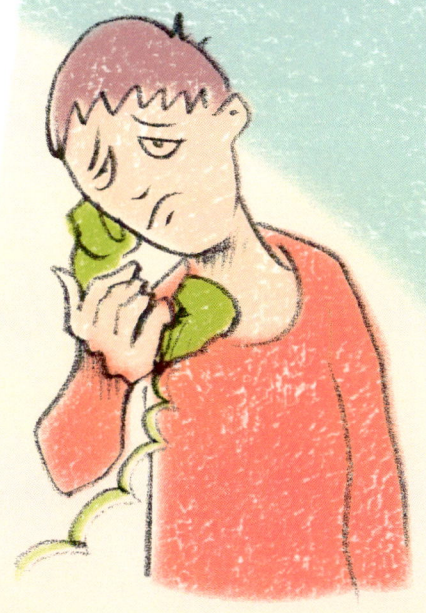

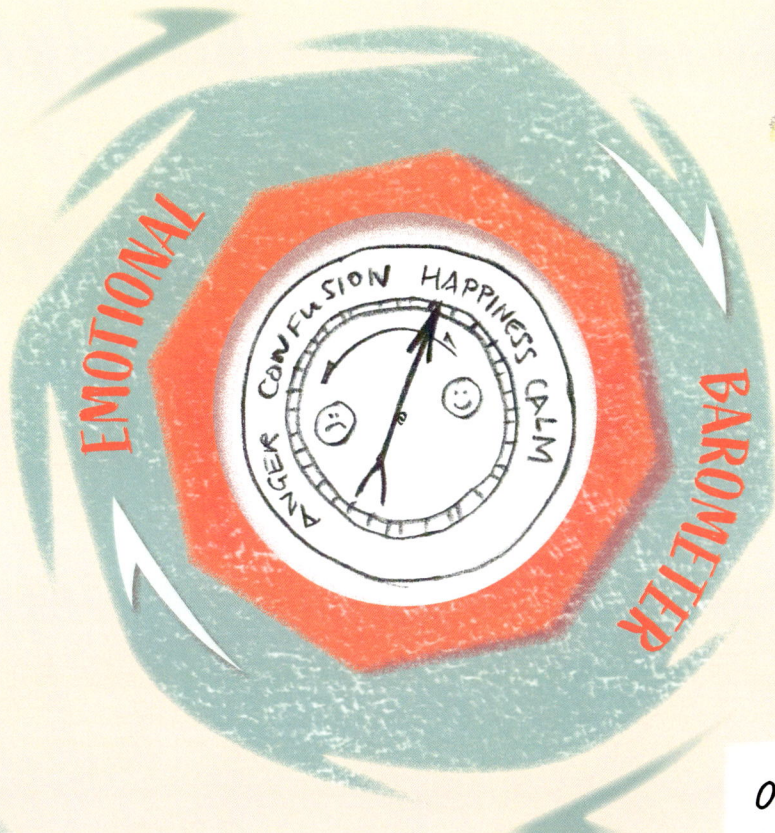

EMOTIONAL BAROMETER

Our voice is like a *barometer*, responding to how we are feeling, and communicating that with our outside world.

21

Our ability to do this is the result of the way the whole system, including our breathing, nervous system, and brain, interacts.

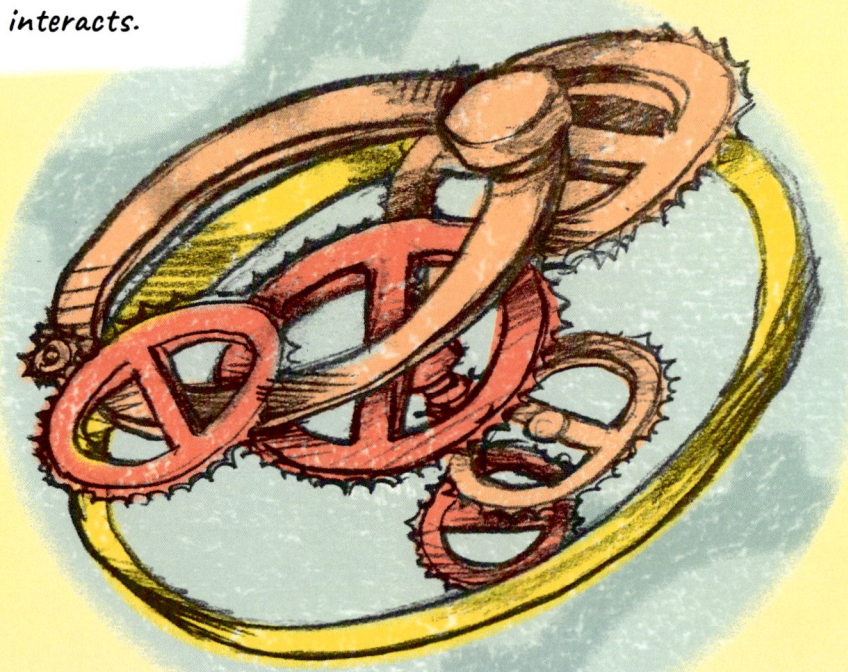

When we talk about the voice, or any system in the body, we are referencing just one part of a whole mind-body experience. In other words *a whole person with unique biopsychosocial factors*. No system, or symptom, exists in a vacuum.

We can think of this system like an intricate, integrated mechanism — a bit like the inner workings of a clock.

All the individual parts need to work together *in harmony* for optimal function.

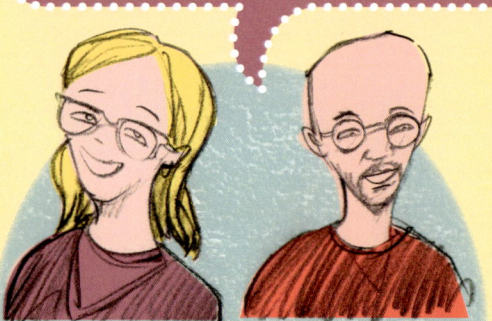

The face of a clock shows us the time, in the same way that our voice shows us *the end result of an internal system*.

If something goes wrong at any point in the system, this can have *ripple effects* all the way through the mechanism, and change the way the muscles in our throat are working.

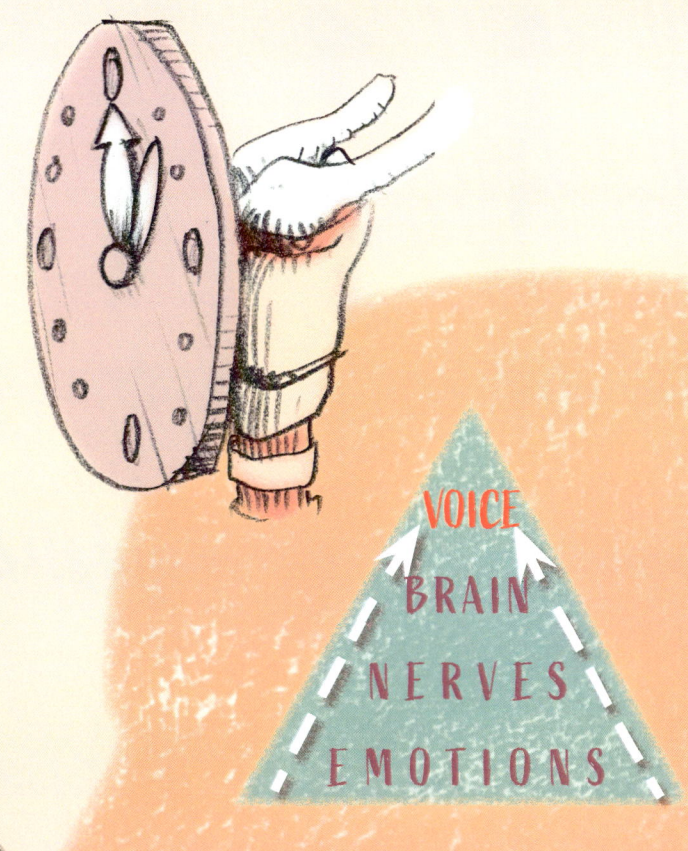

VOICE
BRAIN
NERVES
EMOTIONS

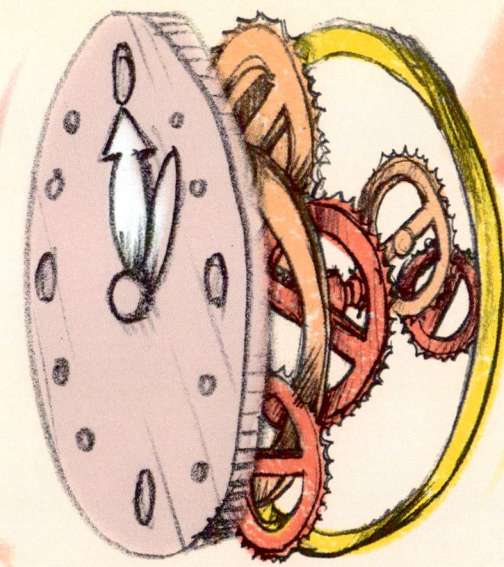

Another 'output' for this system is our breathing. Our breathing has a *direct link* to our nervous system, and when we are under stress, our breathing pattern will change.

The reverse also occurs – if our breathing pattern is not optimal, this is very likely to trigger the stress response in the body.

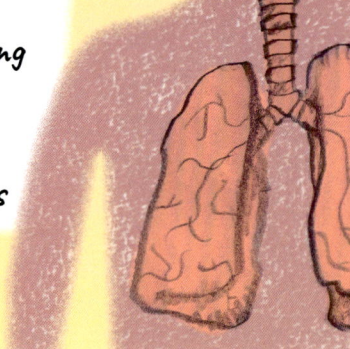

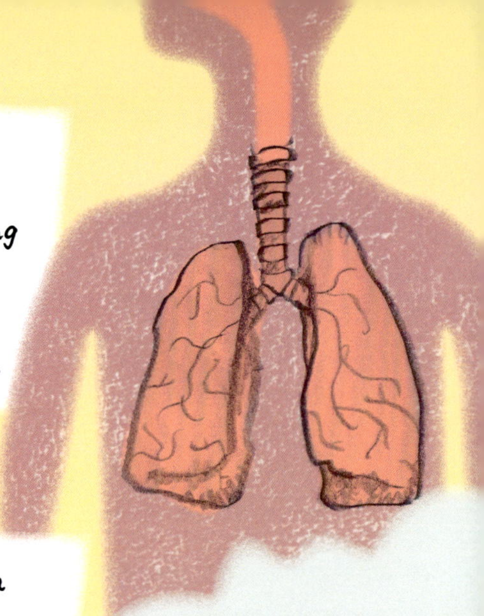

Breathing fast in a 'shallow' way triggers the *sympathetic* branch of the nervous system – this is our *'fight flight'* response.

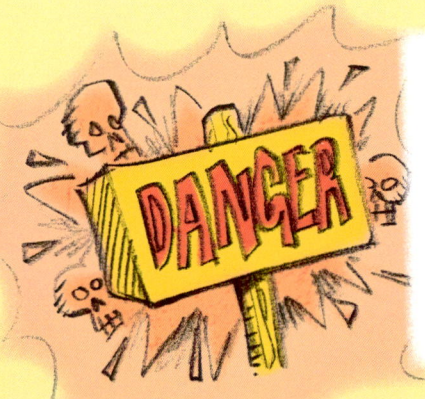

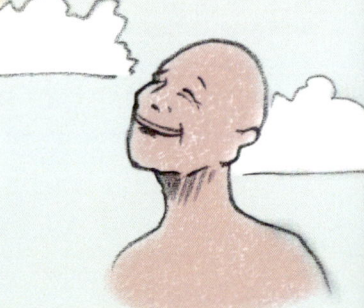

Breathing to the base of the lungs using the diaphragm activates the *parasympathetic** branch of the nervous system. This is the *'rest and digest'* state, which calms us *down*.

We'll talk more about breathing later...

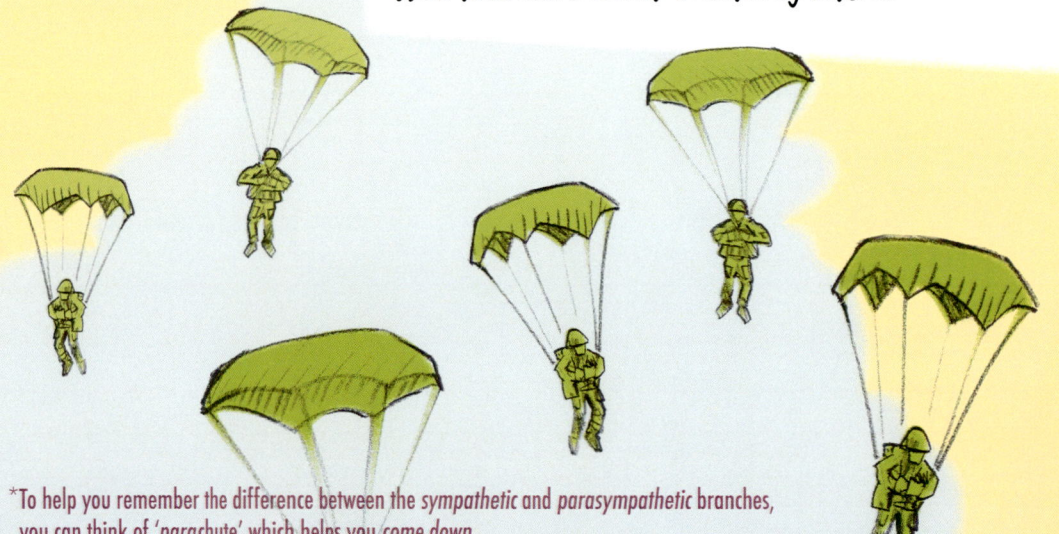

*To help you remember the difference between the *sympathetic* and *parasympathetic* branches, you can think of *'parachute'* which helps you *come down*.

When the vocal mechanism is disrupted, and the muscles start working differently, the system can become 'stuck'.

It can be difficult for this process to reverse on its own...

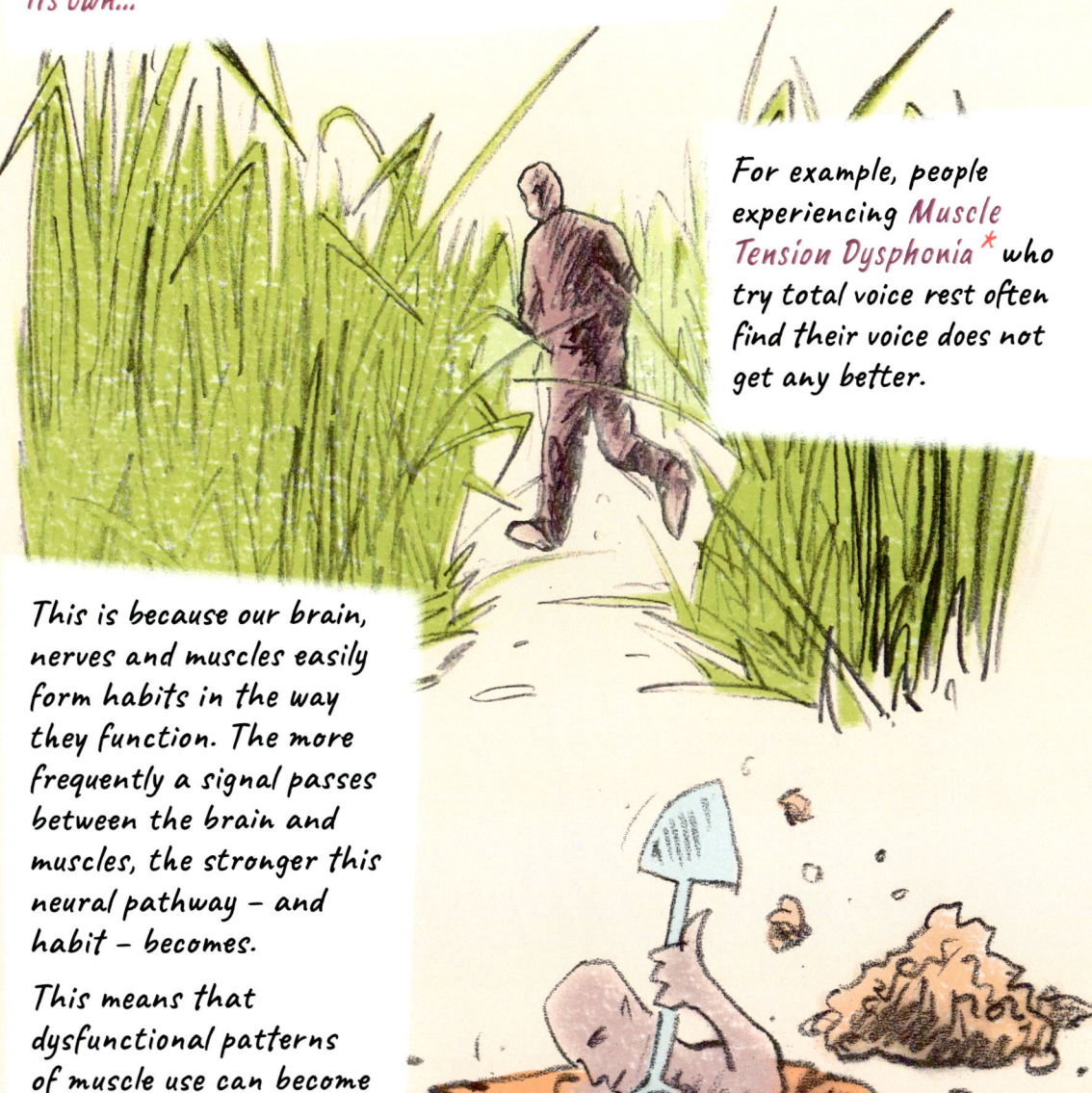

For example, people experiencing *Muscle Tension Dysphonia**** who try total voice rest often find their voice does not get any better.

This is because our brain, nerves and muscles easily form habits in the way they function. The more frequently a signal passes between the brain and muscles, the stronger this neural pathway – and habit – becomes.

This means that dysfunctional patterns of muscle use can become 'entrenched', and the longer they exist, the more 'stuck' they become.

*Don't worry about this term – we'll come back to it later in the book.

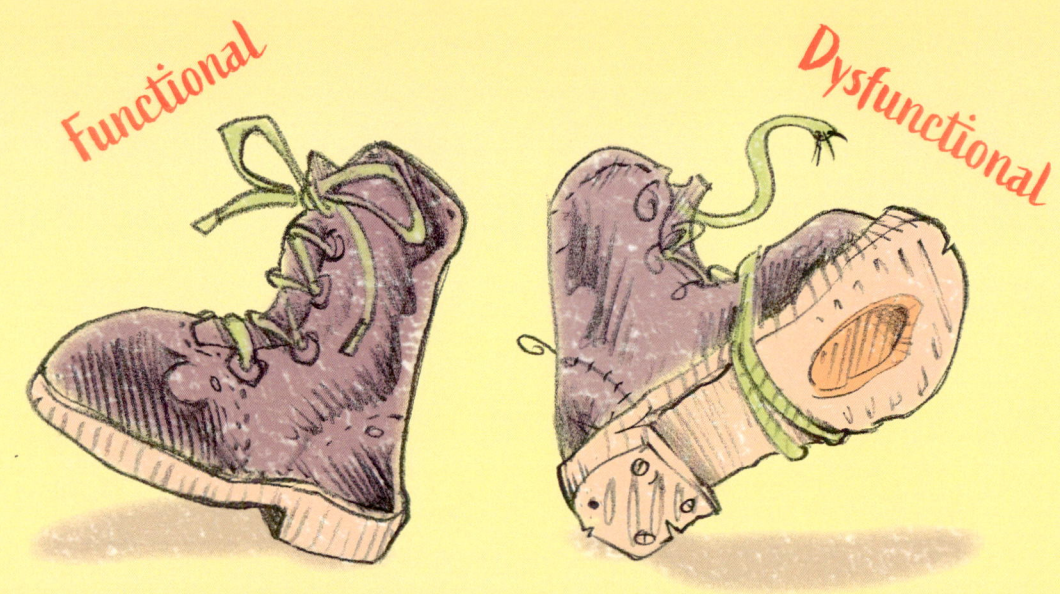

Functional   *Dysfunctional*

What is this telling me?

We have attachments to the way we do things, and it can be interesting to reflect on this in the context of a voice problem.

When we develop dysfunctional patterns, we can think about whether they have a role or purpose in our life. The dysfunction might be telling us we are acting in a way that is *biomechanically*, *psychologically* or *socially* detrimental. Or, it may be that we are internalising messages we are receiving from other people, such as 'I should be seen and not heard', and this is changing the way we behave.

The way we relate to our habits is important, and can help, or hinder, our recovery.

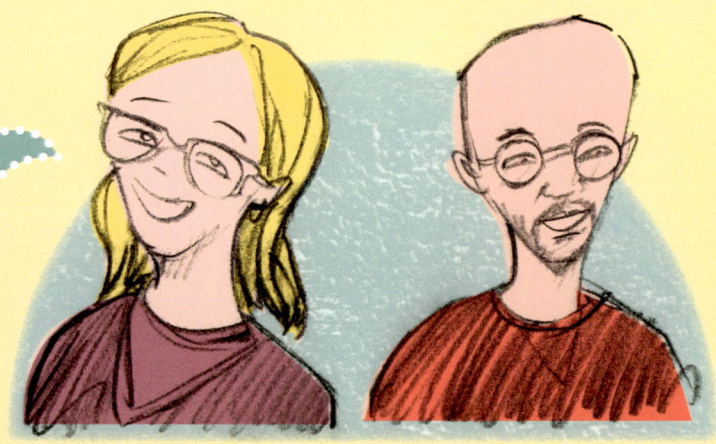

Simply put, the symptoms you experience are your body sending you a message.

We are wired to survive. Because of this, when we perceive a threat (which for early humans would be genuinely life-threatening, and for modern humans might be a triggering email from your boss), our nervous system is *primed to react* in our best interests for survival.

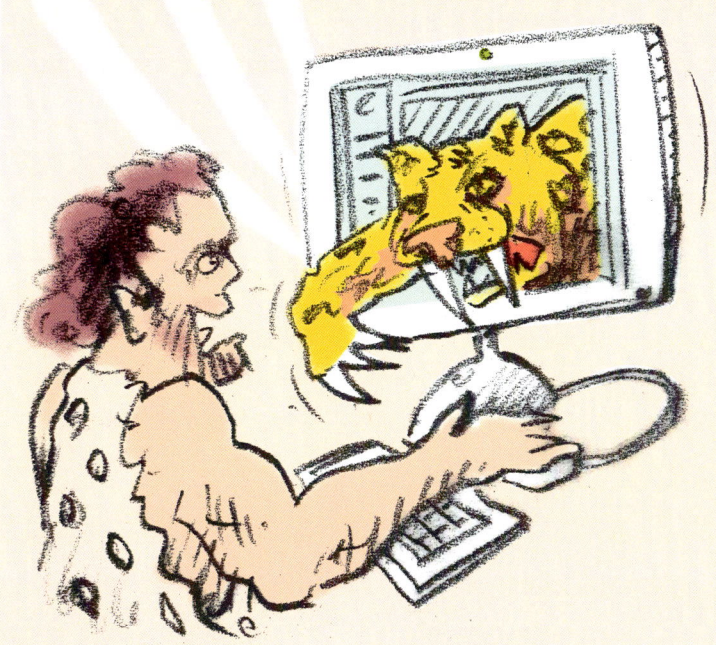

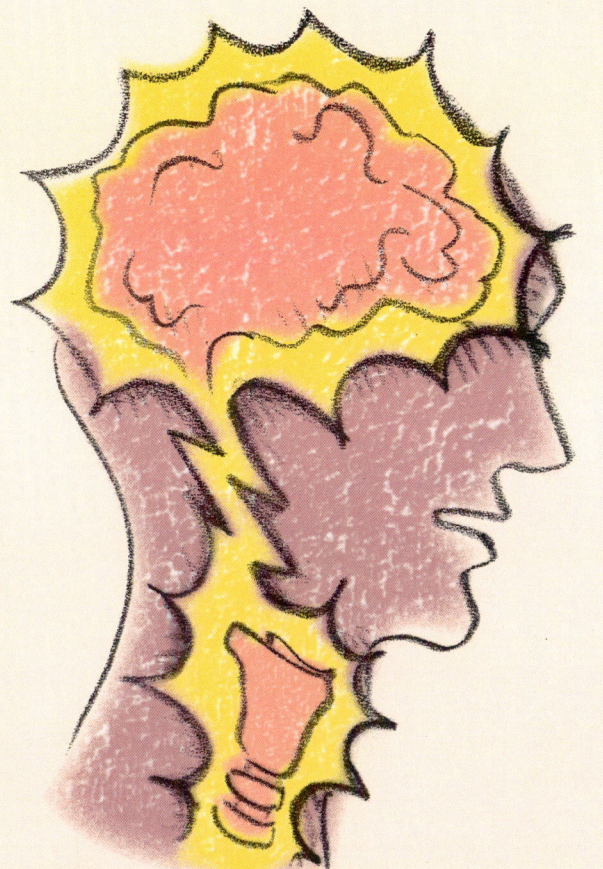

If you are experiencing long-term throat pain or discomfort, although this may feel localised to a particular area, it is often a result of a *wider dysfunction of your nervous system*.

It is the same process as in other forms of chronic pain[*].

* Book recommendation: 'Pain Is Really Strange' by Steve Haines

Your environment, and the people in it, will influence you (and your nervous system) positively or negatively. This impact on the nervous system can filter through the system to your voice.

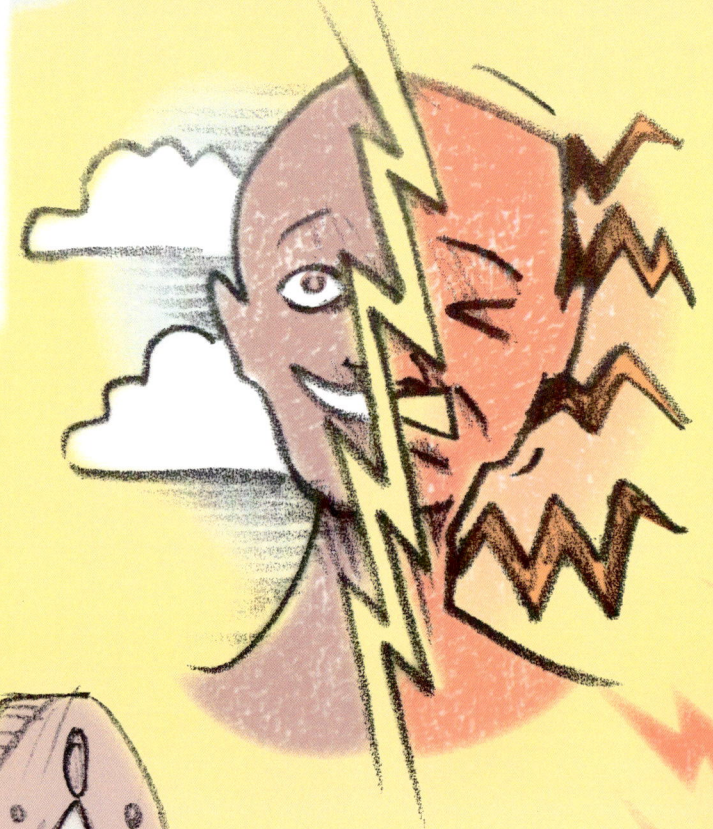

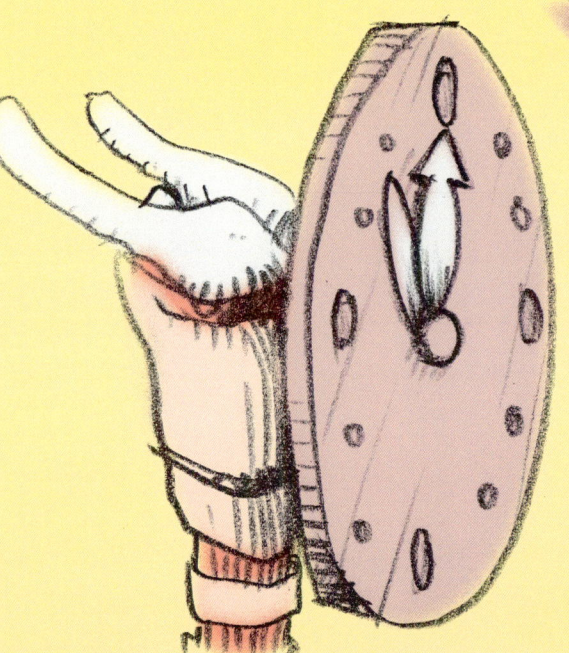

Living in a prolonged state of stress or anxiety*, will usually make throat symptoms worse, and in some cases can be the sole cause of dysfunction.

*This could be a single traumatic event, or a prolonged period of difficult circumstances.

"Let's return to our pathway to recovery"

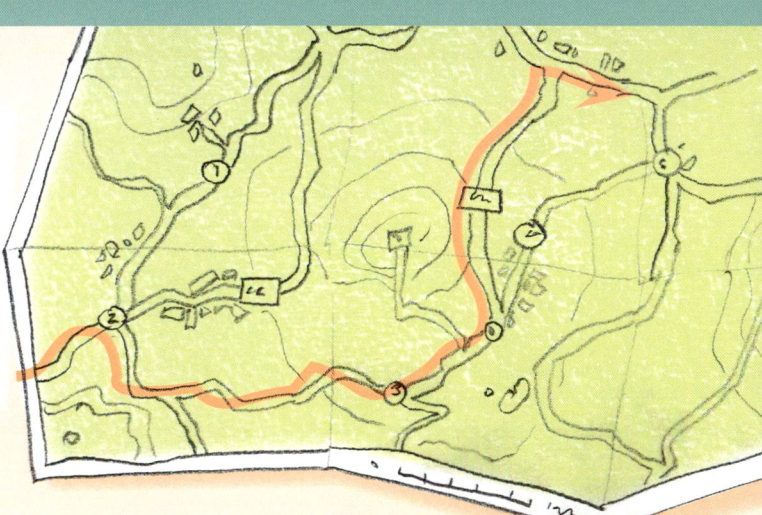

Now that we have explored some of the systems that influence our voices, let's return to our pathway to recovery...

If your GP feels you need more specialist medical care, or if they have been unable to help, they should refer you to an *Ear, Nose and Throat (ENT)* doctor.

The ideal place to be seen is a *Joint Voice Clinic*, which is a specialist voice clinic run by a laryngologist (voice specialist) and speech therapist.

There may not be a clinic in your local area, although if you are a professional voice user your GP should consider *referring you further afield*, for example to a performing arts specialist.

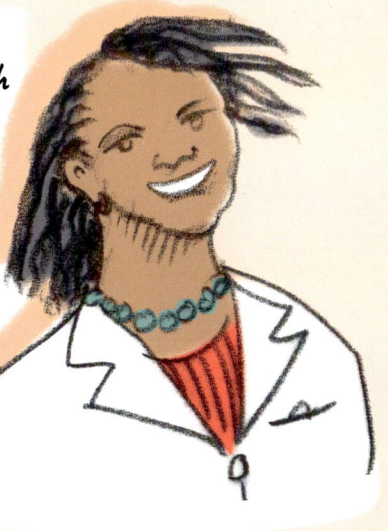
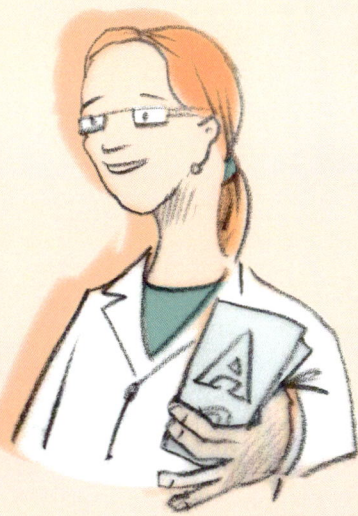

At your ENT appointment, your vocal tract will be examined using a camera, usually via a flexible nasendoscopy (through your nose). This is called a laryngoscopy.

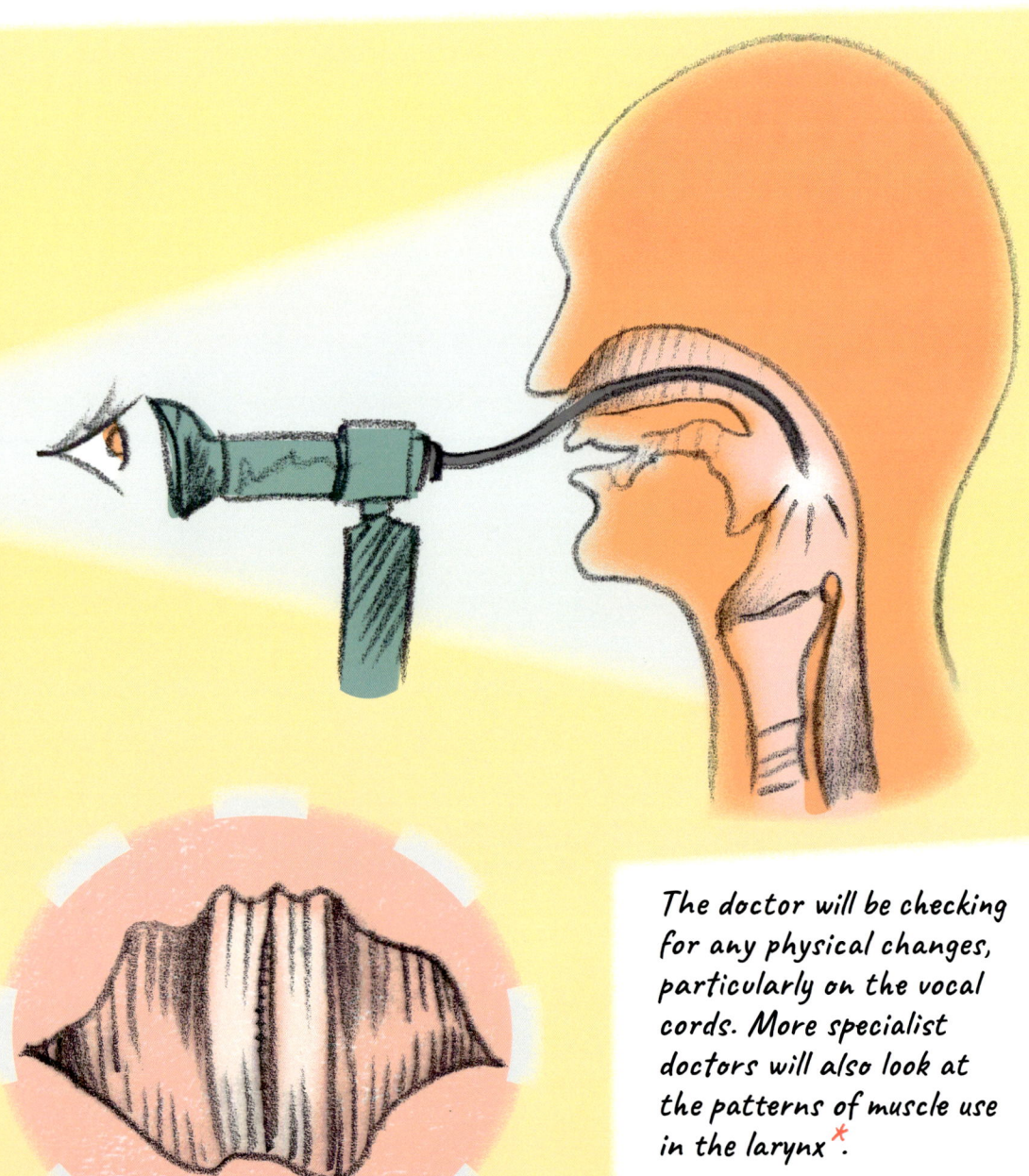

The doctor will be checking for any physical changes, particularly on the vocal cords. More specialist doctors will also look at the patterns of muscle use in the larynx*.

*You should ask your ENT doctor if they can provide images from your nasendoscopy for you. If you are being seen by a voice specialist, their equipment should easily make this possible.

The diagnosis you are given by the ENT doctor will generally fall into one of two categories:

Structural
Where there is a physical abnormality

or

Functional
Where the mechanism itself appears healthy, but the action is suboptimal

Structural conditions:

These include *'lumps and bumps'* on the vocal cords like:
- nodules, polyps and cysts
- changes to the tissues such as inflammation and oedema (swelling)
- or reduced movement of the vocal cords caused by nerve damage.

Functional conditions:

These are usually described as *muscle tension dysphonia* (MTD).

MTD is when the muscles of the larynx lose coordination, and don't work well. Dysphonia literally means voice (phonia) problem (dys). When combined with muscle tension, this can lead to symptoms of vocal strain, fatigue, hoarseness, voice loss and pain.

Often *structural* and *functional* conditions occur together.

Other functional conditions include...

Globus (a feeling of a lump in your throat or something stuck), some forms of *Dysphagia* (difficulty swallowing), and certain types of *cough* and *breathing difficulties**

These conditions fall under the umbrella of *hypersensitivity*.
- Hypersensitivity involves the nerves of the throat becoming oversensitive and hyperreactive.
- This alters the signals sent to and from your brain.

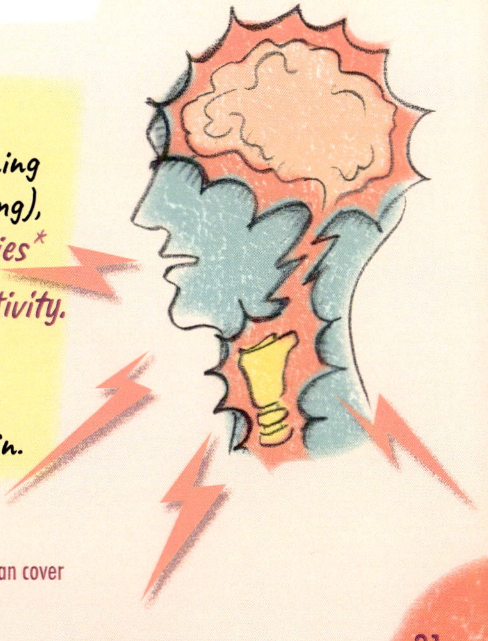

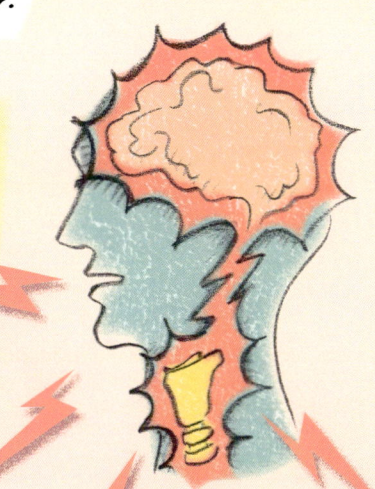

*These particular symptoms are complex and require a deeper dive than this book can cover

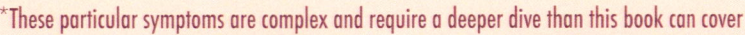

Sometimes, you may come away from an ENT appointment feeling like you have not been given a clear diagnosis. If there are no structural abnormalities, it may seem like you have been told that 'there is nothing wrong'.

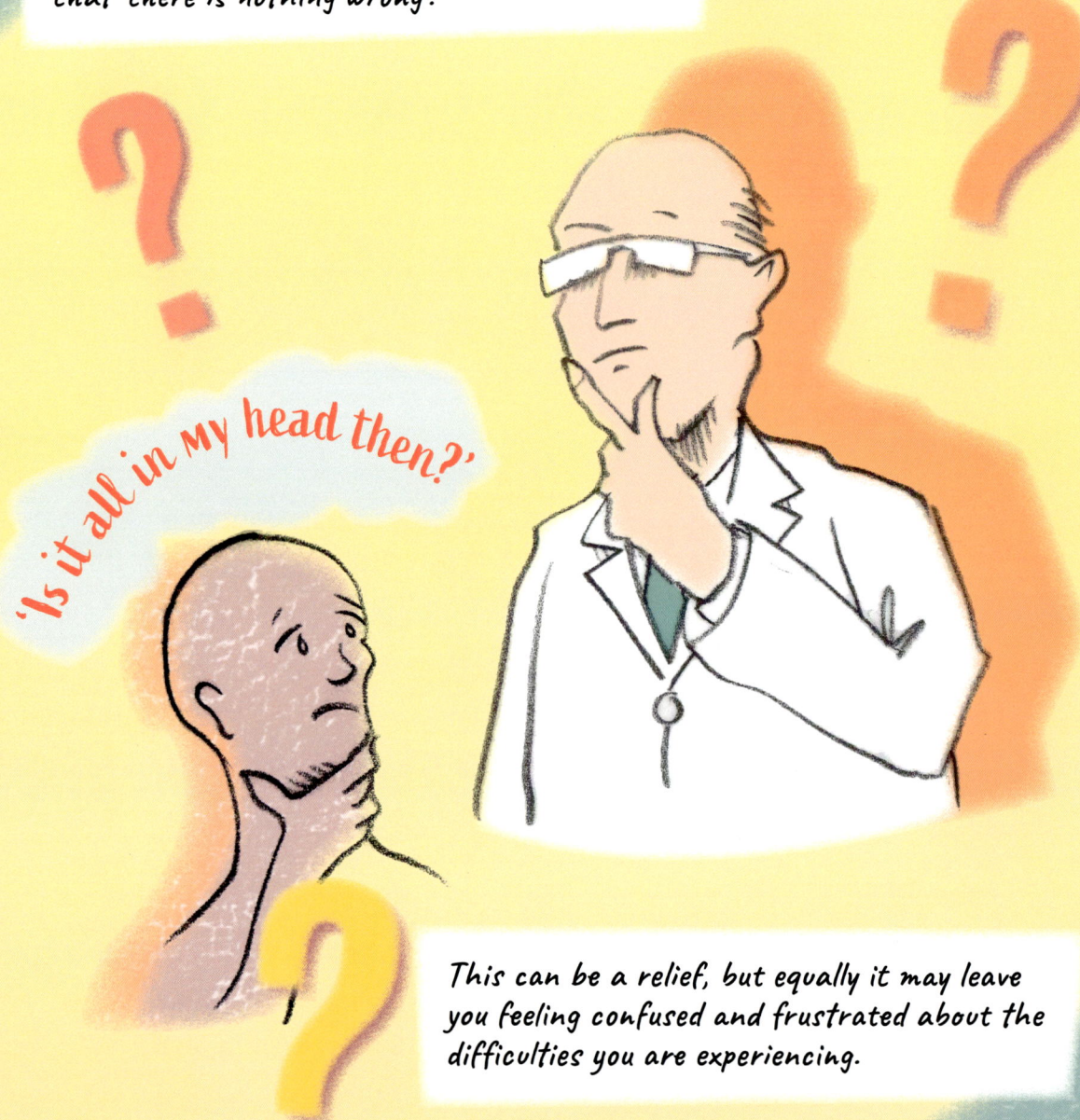

'Is it all in my head then?'

This can be a relief, but equally it may leave you feeling confused and frustrated about the difficulties you are experiencing.

The treatment you are recommended will depend on the underlying nature of your voice or throat problem.

Generally, if there is a structural problem, surgery may be needed at some point to fully restore your voice - your ENT doctor will advise on this.

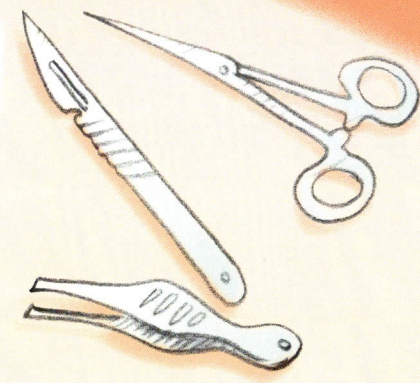

For functional problems, treatment is likely to involve therapy or rehabilitation. (Of course this is also an important element in treating structural conditions)

BUT... as we know, the voice is truly *bio-psycho-social* and, most of the time, healing and recovery require care that transcends the biomedical model. This is not a new concept and is where biopsychosocial medicine comes in.

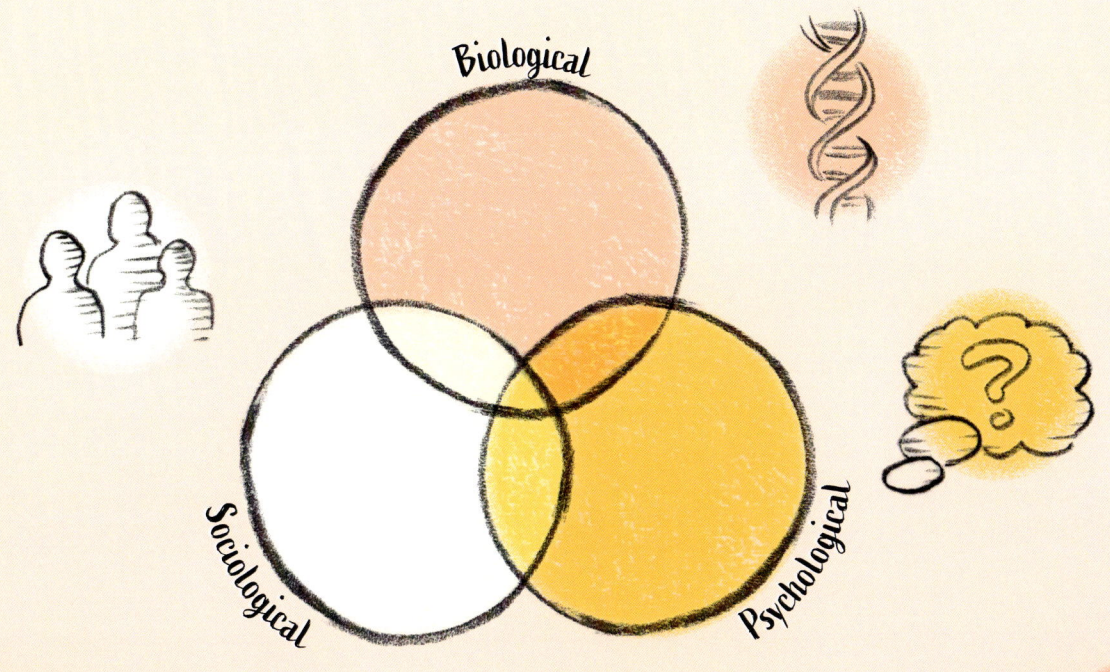

Most people benefit from a referral to a voice specialist *Speech and Language Therapist* (SLT). This is because, generally speaking, ENT doctors specialise in biomedical aspects of the voice, i.e. what can be treated with medications and surgery. An SLT will spend more time exploring the psychosocial aspects of symptoms.

There are many other people that may help you on your path, and working with a multidisciplinary team will optimise your recovery.

This team may include...

- a singing teacher or voice coach, ideally a voice rehabilitation specialist — this is very important if you are a singer
- a counsellor or psychotherapist
- a mindfulness or mindset coach
- a nutritionist
- an exercise coach or personal trainer
- a manual therapist such as an osteopath or massage therapist
- and most importantly... **you!**

YOU are the most important person in your journey. Because the voice is so intricately connected to our internal and external world, it is not necessarily something that can be 'fixed' by other people alone (although the skills of specialists are important).

Equally important are your own *mindset*, *motivation* and *acceptance*.

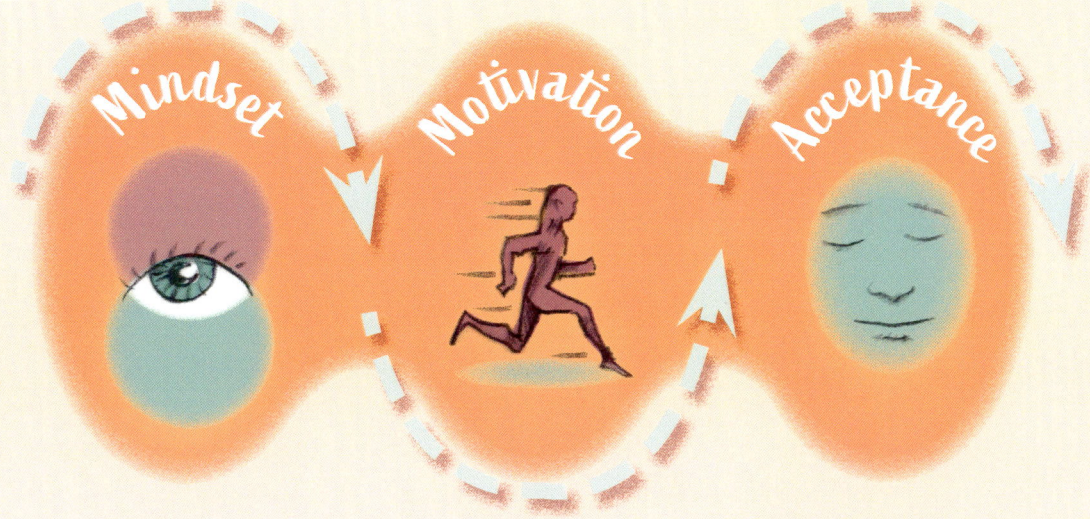

Let's explore some of the ways that you can be the partner, rather than the patient, in your health and wellness.

"So what can I do to help myself?"

"So, what can I do to help myself before I get to see a specialist?"

Rest your voice, but not too much

You want to reduce any inflammation in the vocal cords with periodic resting. Think of your voice as a phone battery which may need to be put 'on charge' or 'on airplane' mode at times.

> **DISCLAIMER:**
> Whilst these suggestions below are safe, there may be some conditions or symptoms which are exacerbated by doing any one of these. Again, we encourage you to own your recovery, which means **if it doesn't feel helpful, stop.**

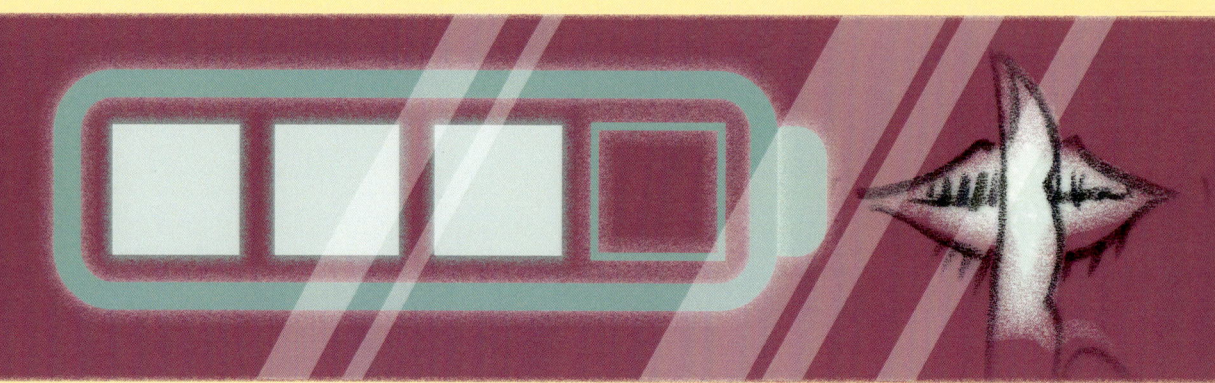

Keep your voice gently moving

Speaking and doing gentle voice exercises, like straw phonation, are important to keep the muscles of your voice moving and stretching. Avoid things that feel like they are putting too much pressure on your voice, and rest your voice if it feels tired, sore or strained.

Straw phonation involves putting a straw (ideally a reusable one) into a small amount of water and blowing bubbles. You can do this whilst making sound, or silently. This increases air pressure in the vocal tract, which has a 'cushioning' effect for the vocal cords.

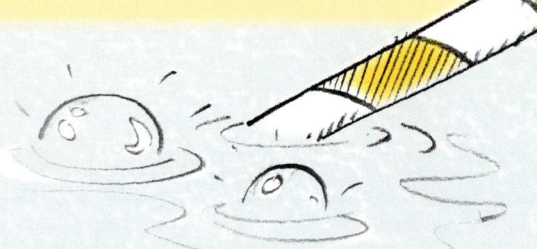

Take a breath

Do you remember when we mentioned how breathing can activate the *sympathetic* (stress) or *parasympathetic* (rest) branches of the nervous system? Practising *slow diaphragmatic breathing* (think of breathing down to your belly), *through your nose*, can quickly help to balance your physical and mental state*.

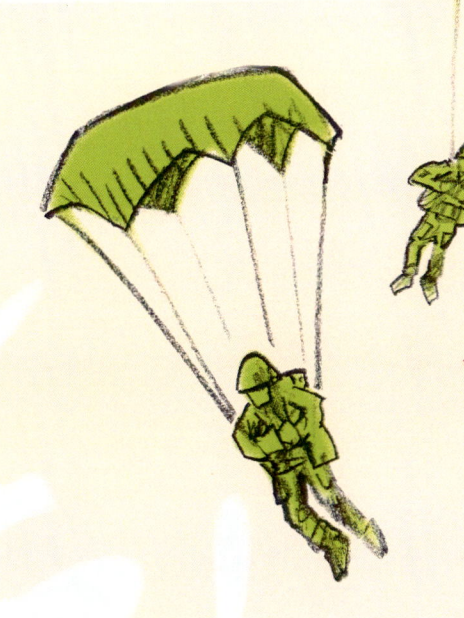

*If you are interested in learning more about breathing, look up 'Breath' by James Nestor.

Drink plenty of water

Staying well hydrated is one of the simplest and most important ways to look after your voice. It helps to keep your vocal cords lubricated and supple. Good hydration§ should be continuous, so *sip regularly through the day* – try to make sure you drink something every hour.

§The current research suggests drinking 1ml of water for every calorie burned during the day. For example, if you burn 1800 calories, you should aim to drink 1.8 litres of water. You know when you are adequately hydrated when your wee is a pale colour.

Get a change of scene, preferably in nature.

Getting out of your immediate environment can be really beneficial for your overall health, especially somewhere you can see the horizon. If you remember earlier, we looked at how our brain perceives threat. If we can see the horizon, our primal brain can determine whether there are any threats to our life about!

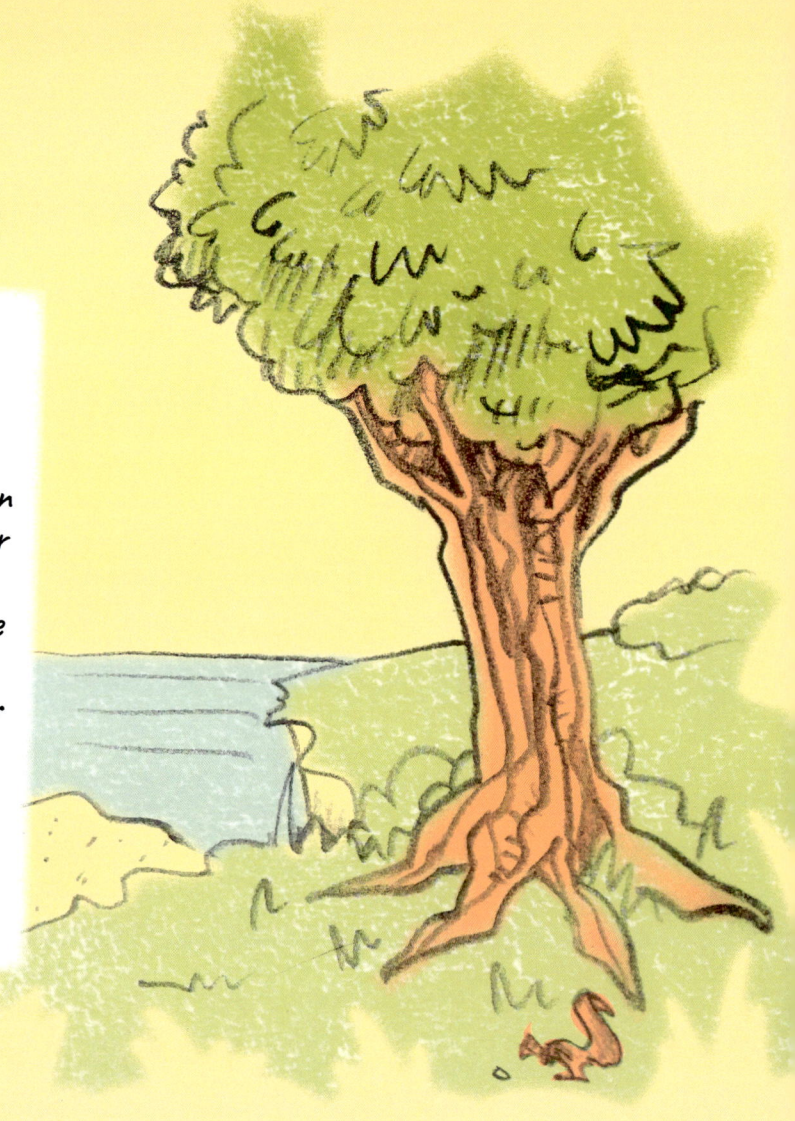

Doing this can help you feel more *biopsychosocially* safe.

See a specialist such as those we mentioned earlier.

Even just booking an appointment with a specialist can ease your symptoms, as you have taken *active steps* in your healing and recovery.

It is helpful to increase your awareness of your overall health and wellbeing.

Ask yourself questions like these...

How often do I move my body?*

Is the food I eat nourishing me?

Am I prioritising my self care?

Do I get enough sleep?

*This doesn't have to be grand or intensive, but the World Health Organisation recommend you should do at least 150-300 minutes of moderate-intensity, or 75-150 minutes of vigorous-intensity, aerobic physical activity, (or an equivalent combination) throughout the week.

Now that we are reaching the end of this book, we hope you feel like you have a *better understanding* about how your voice works, what can go wrong, and the importance of biopsychosocial treatment and care.

YOU steer the ship in your vocal recovery, so it is important that you feel *listened to* when you seek out a specialist to guide you on your journey.

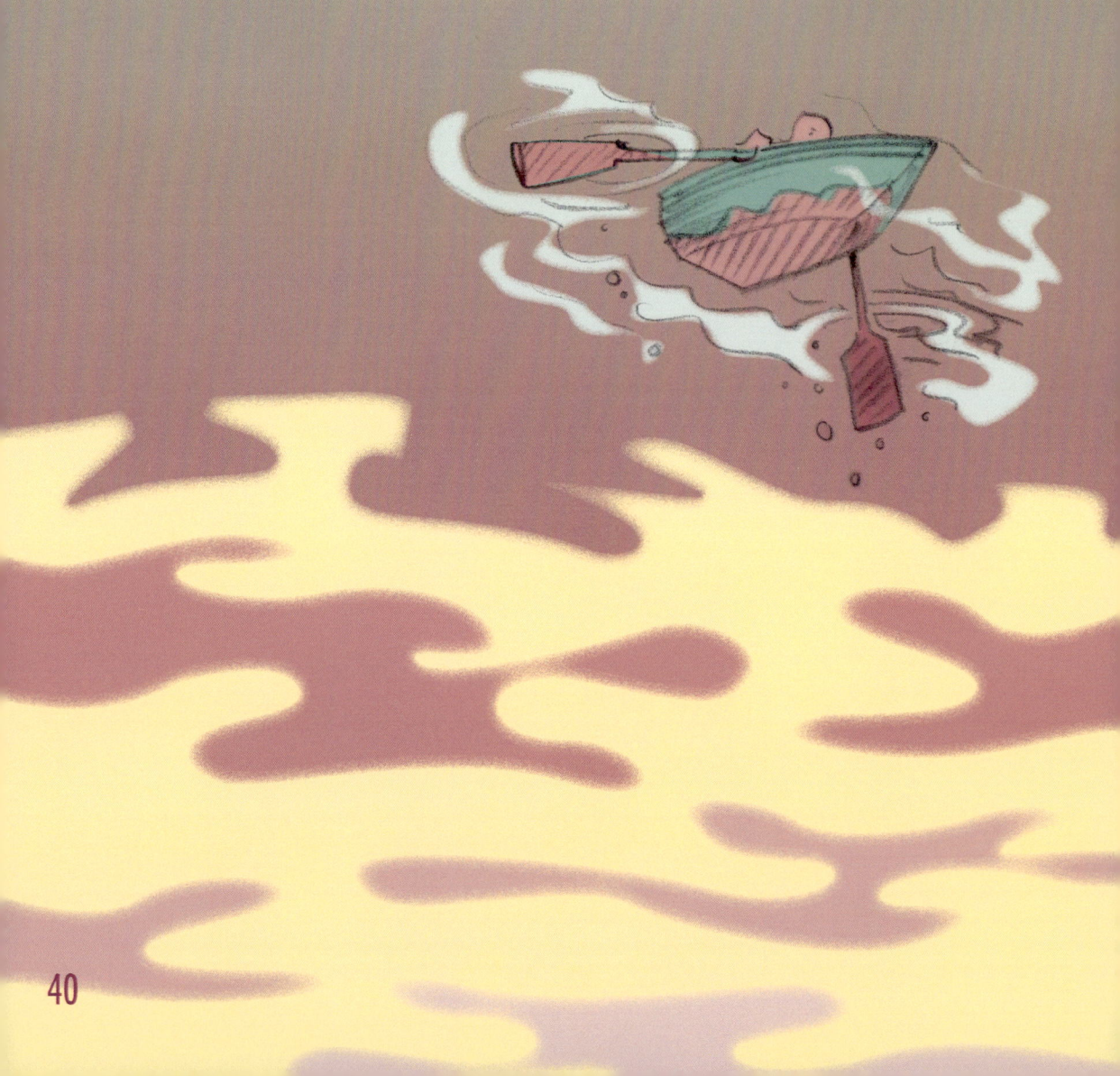

The voice is complex and usually there are multiple factors influencing the problem that has developed. Optimal recovery usually needs each of these areas to be explored, like different pieces of a puzzle.

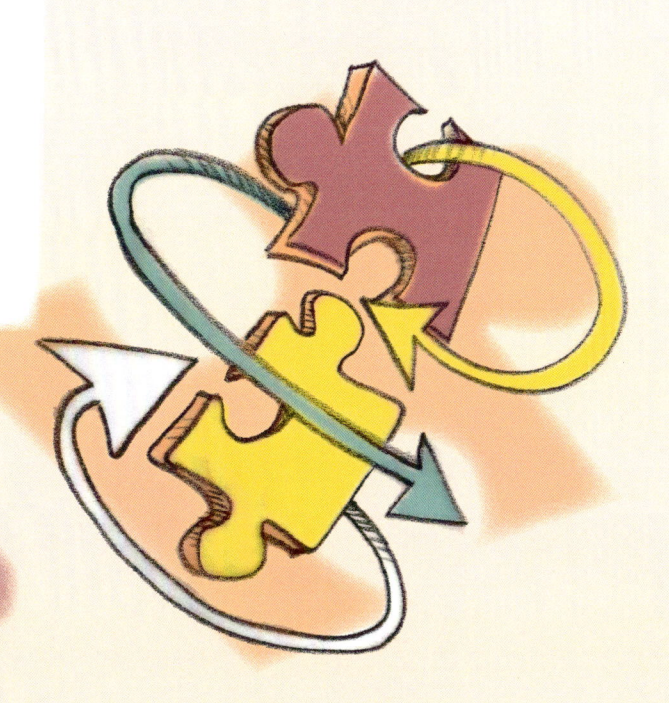

The nervous system, if overloaded by stress, can be susceptible to 'misfiring'. This is particularly relevant when there is a trigger, like a viral infection, which sets the body into dysfunctional patterns*.

*This explains why our symptoms can seem to appear 'out of the blue' – it can be likened to 'the straw that broke the camel's back'.

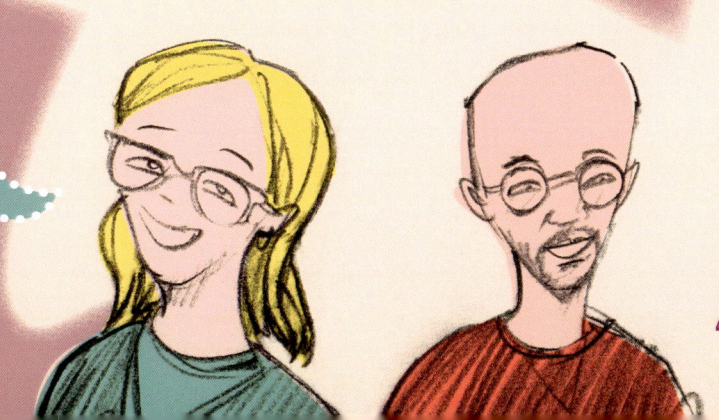

When dealing with a voice problem, it is important to think about *all aspects of your life*, and not just what might be happening with your vocal cords.

Our voices are a huge part of our identity. Having a problem with your voice can be scary, affecting your work and social life, and even how you feel about yourself.

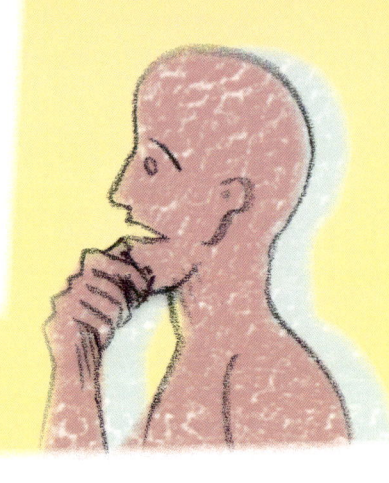

But *you aren't alone*, and by empowering yourself with knowledge, and finding the right specialists, you are taking the steps you need to not only recover, but to optimise your vocal health for the future.

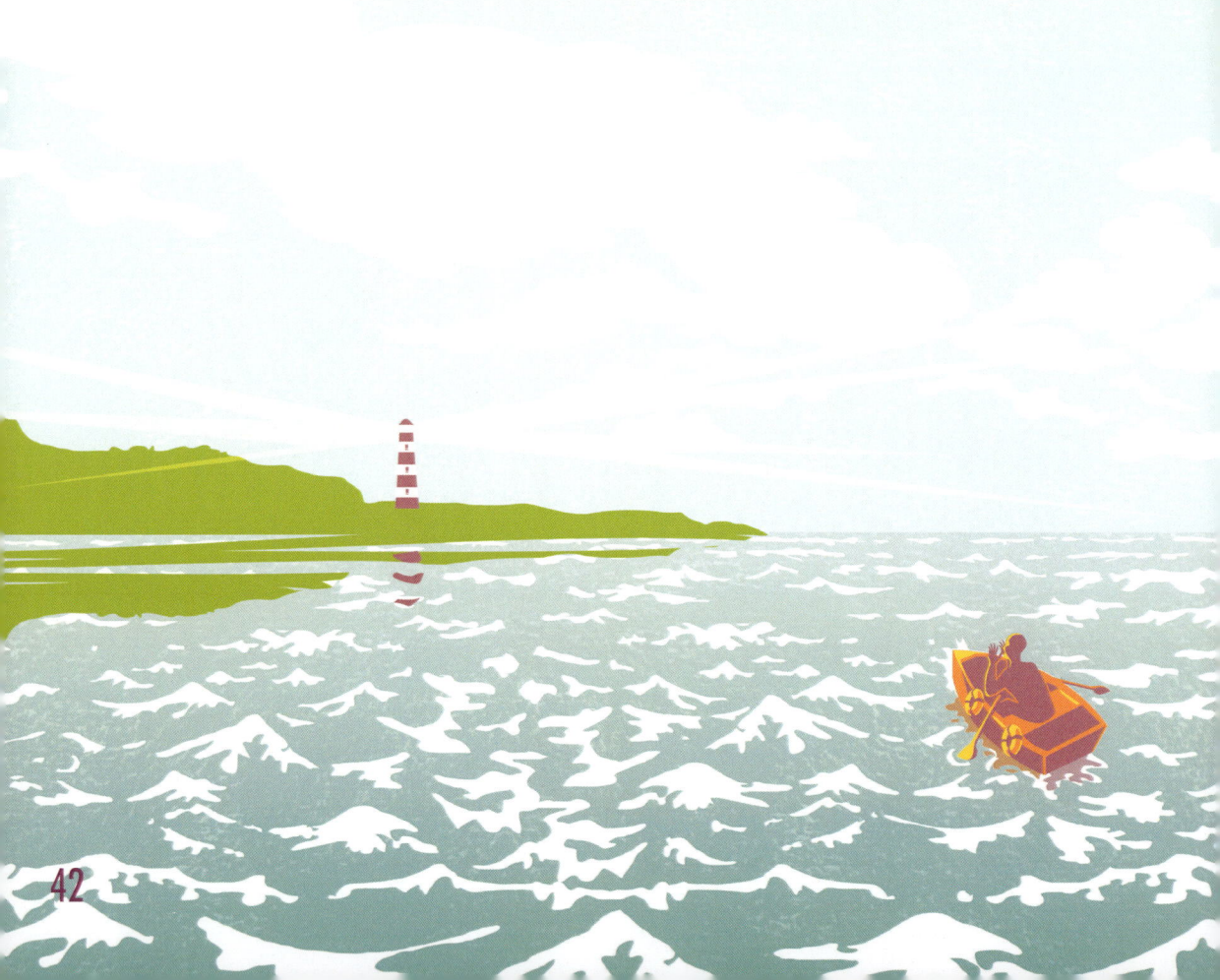

At the heart of this book is a message of hope.

If you are a person experiencing a voice problem, we hope that this book has given you some insight and empowerment to move forward in your journey.

If you are a professional working in this field, we hope that this book will be useful for the people you are working with.

Thank you for being a part of our quest to give everyone a voice.

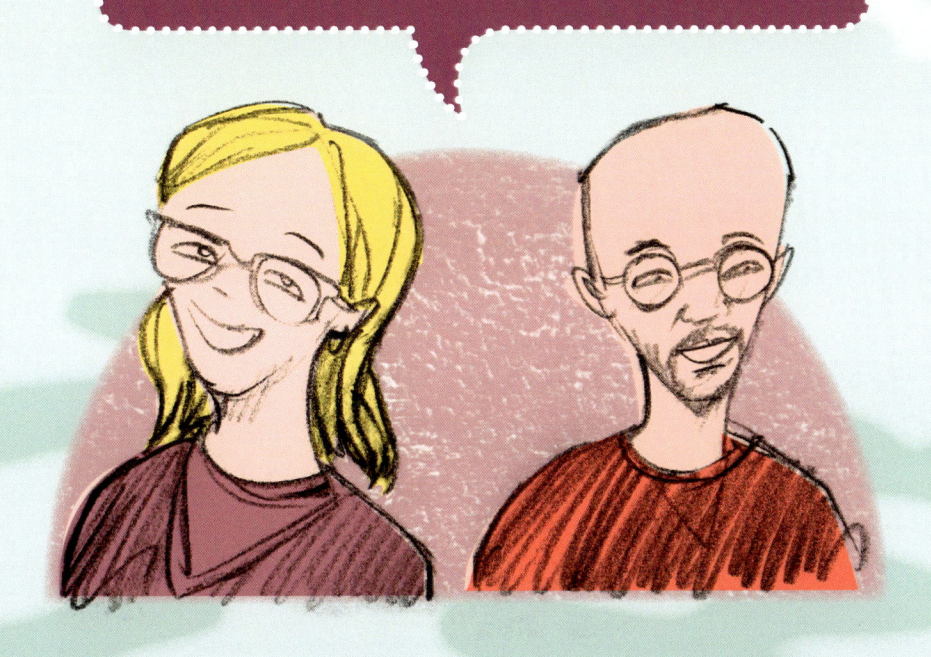

REFERENCES

Anders Ericsson, K., Krampe, R. and Tesch-Romer, C. (1993) The role of deliberate practice in the acquisition of expert performance. *Psychological Review* 100:363–406.

Bunch Dayme, M. (2009) *Dynamics of the Singing Voice*, 5th edn. Vienna & New York, NY: Springer.

Cancer Research UK (2021) Cancer Survival Statistics [online]. Available at: https://www.cancerresearchuk.org/health-professional/cancerstatistics/survival [Accessed 16 November 2021].

Cohen, S.M., Kim, J., Roy, N., *et al.* (2012) Prevalence and causes of dysphonia in a large treatment-seeking population. *Laryngoscope* 122(2):343–8. doi: 10.1002/lary.22426. PMID: 22271658.

Cohen, S.M., Dinan, M.A., Roy, N., *et al.* (2014) Diagnosis change in voice-disordered patients evaluated by primary care and/or otolaryngology: A longitudinal study. *Otolaryngology-Head & Neck Surgery* 150:95–102.

Chitnis, A., Dowrick, C., Byng, R., & Turner, P.D.S. (2011) *Guidance for Health Professionals on Medically Unexplained Symptoms* London: Royal College of General Practitioners.

Engel, G.L. (1977) The need for a new medical model: A challenge for biomedicine. *Science* 196(4286):129–36. https://doi.org/10.1126/science. 847460.

Eriksen, T.E., Kerry, R., Mumford, S., *et al.* (2013) At the borders of medical reasoning: Aetiological and ontological challenges of medically unexplained symptoms. *Philosophy, Ethics, and Humanities in Medicine* 8:11. https://doi.org/10.1186/1747-5341-8-11.

Greenhalgh, T., Howick, J. & Maskrey, N. (2014) Evidence based medicine: A movement in crisis? *British Medical Journal* 348:g3725–g3725.

Haines, S. (2015) *Pain Is Really Strange* London: Singing Dragon.

Howard, D.M. (1998) Practical voice measurement. In: Harris, T. *et al.* (eds) *The Voice Clinic Handbook*, pp.323–380. London: Whurr.

Jung, S., Park, H., Bae, H., *et al.* (2016) Laryngeal myofascial pain syndrome as a new diagnostic entity of dysphonia Department of Otorhinolaryngology - Head and Neck Surgery, Ewha Womans University School of Medicine.

Karkos, P.D., Thomas, L., Temple, R.H. & Issing, W.J. (2005) Awareness of general practitioners towards treatment of laryngopharyngeal reflux: A British Survey, *Journal of Otolaryngology-Head & Neck Surgery* 133(4):505–8.

Mathieson, L. (2011) The evidence for laryngeal manual therapies in the treatment of muscle tension dysphonia. *Current Opinion in Otolaryngology & Head and Neck Surgery* 19(3):171–6.

Nestor, J. (2020) *Breath: The New Science of a Lost Art* London: Penguin Life.

O'Hara, J., Stocken, D., Watson, G., *et al.* (2021) Use of proton pump inhibitors to treat persistent throat symptoms: multicentre, double blind, randomised, placebo controlled trial. *British Medical Journal* 372:m4903.

Porges, S. (2011) *The Polyvagal Theory: Neurophysiological Foundations of Emotions, Attachment, Communication, and Self-regulation* New York, NY: W.W. Norton.

Reiter, R., Hoffmann, T.K., Pickhard, A. & Brosch, S. (2015) Hoarseness-causes and treatments. *Deutsches Ärzteblatt international* 112(19):329–37. doi:10.3238/arztebl.2015.0329.

Rogers, C. (1961) *On Becoming a Person: A Therapist's View of Psychotherapy* London: Constable.

Sama, A., Carding, P.N., Price, S., *et al.* (2001) The clinical features of functional dysphonia. *Laryngoscope* 111(3):458–63.

Schneider, C.M. & Dennehy, K.G. (1997) Exercise physiology principles applied to vocal performance: The improvement of postural alignment. *Journal of Voice* 11(3):332–7.

Steinbrecher, N., Koerber, S., Frieser, D. & Hiller, W. (2011) The prevalence of medically unexplained symptoms in primary care. *Psychosomatics* 52(3):263–71. 10.1016/j.psym.2011.01.007.

Testa, M. & Rossettini, G. (2016) Enhance placebo, avoid nocebo: How contextual factors affect physiotherapy outcomes. *Manual Therapy* 24:65–74. http://dx.doi.org/10.1016/j.math.2016.04.006.

Thompson, W.G. & Heaton, K.W. (1982) Heartburn and globus in apparently healthy people. *Canadian Medical Association Journal* 126(1):46–8.

Copyright © Lydia Hart & Stephen R King 2022

Art and design by Stewart Harris

All rights reserved. No part of this publication may be reproduced or transmitted in any form or by any means, electronic or mechanical including photocopying recording or by any information and storage retrieval system, without prior written consent from the publisher.

This is a first edition.

Published by New Voice Publishing.

www.newvoicepublishing.co.uk

ISBN 978-1-3999-3307-0

Printed and bound in Great Britain.

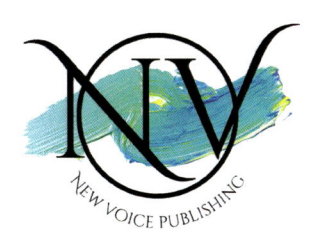